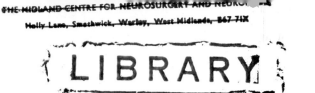
STATISTICAL METHODS IN MEDICAL INVESTIGATIONS

Second Edition

To Mary-Elizabeth

STATISTICAL METHODS IN MEDICAL INVESTIGATIONS

Second Edition

Brian S Everitt
Professor of Statistics in Behavioural Science
Institute of Psychiatry, London

Edward Arnold
A member of the Hodder Headline Group
LONDON MELBOURNE AUCKLAND

Copublished in the Americas by Halsted Press
an imprint of John Wiley & Sons Inc.
New York — Toronto

© 1994 B. S. Everitt

First published in Great Britain 1989
Second edition 1994

Copublished in the Americas by Halsted Press, an imprint of John
Wiley & Sons, Inc., 605 Third Avenue, New York, NY10158

British Library Cataloguing in Publication Data

Everitt, Brian
  Statistical Methods for Medical
  Investigations. – 2Rev.ed
  I. Title
  610.72

ISBN 0 340 61431 5

Library of Congress Cataloging-in-Publication Data

Available upon request

ISBN 0 470 23383 4

Printed and bound in Great Britain for Edward Arnold, a division of
Hodder Headline PLC, 338 Euston Road, London NW1 3BH
by the University Press, Cambridge

Preface to second edition

The first edition of *Statistical Methods for Medical Investigations* arose from trying to provide a general account of some of the statistical methodology increasingly used in medical research, but not covered in standard texts such as Armitage and Berry (1987) or Altman (1991). The second edition has the same aim and is again directed towards readers who are familiar with common statistical methods such as *t*-tests, chi-square tests, simple regression and the like, and require a fairly concise description of more complex methods, particularly how they might be applied in practice. Consequently this edition, like its predecessor, contains numerous examples, and once again technical details of the methods have been kept relatively brief. But despite these overall similarities, this second edition is considerably different to the first. Each chapter has undergone extensive revision in an attempt to make the material more helpful to those faced with the difficulties of analysing complex medical data. In addition new examples have been added, and topics that in the first edition were not covered or only mentioned in passing, for example, intention-to-treat analysis, meta-analysis, correspondence analysis and missing values, are now covered in more detail. The previous appendix on *Computers and Statistics* has been replaced with a list of relevant statistical software.

Once again I am indebted to researchers at the Institute of Psychiatry who supplied me with data and to publishers and authors who allowed me to reproduce material from their work. I am also grateful to Dr. Graham Dunn and Pak Sham for their helpful comments and suggestions, even the few I have chosen to ignore. Lastly I would like to thank Marie Dyer for typing the manuscript.

B. S. EVERITT
Institute of Psychiatry
September 1993

Contents

1

Statistics in Medicine

1.1 Introduction

A study showing an increase in breast cancer among women who use the pill is likely to spark a new scare when it is released this week.

The study, from Sweden, shows women who use the pill long-term before the age of 25 are at greater risk of the disease later in life...

Another study which contradicts the Swedish findings will be published this week. It will appear in the *British Medical Journal.* It comes from New Zealand, and suggests that the use of the pill is *not* a risk factor in breast cancer.

Researchers in New Zealand can point for support to a vast American study published last month in the *New England Journal of Medicine.* That compared 4711 women with breast cancer to 4670 without the disease and showed no increased risk. It was found that 1756 of those with the disease had used the contraceptive pill while 1699 of those without had also used it. The difference was found to be insignificant in statistical terms.

Observer article, September 1986

Medical research often deals with issues which are of great concern to the general public. Frequently interest lies in the assessment of possible risk factors for some disease. The opening quotation, for example, relates to studies investigating whether or not taking the contraceptive pill is a risk factor for breast cancer. Other examples which have been the subject of considerable debate both in the medical literature and the media in general, are smoking and lung cancer, living close to a nuclear power station and childhood leukaemia, and diet and coronary heart disease.

Of equal importance and concern are studies involved with the evaluation of the therapeutic effects of new treatments, particularly powerful new drugs. Here the consequences of success may be dramatic and alleviate much human suffering (polio vaccine and antibiotics are two examples), but the consequences of errors can be tragic and the cause of much human misery. (The problems with the drug thalidomide illustrates this final point only too dramatically.)

The issues involved in such studies are frequently complex and the effects under investigation relatively subtle, a combination which can lead to different conclusions being reached by workers researching the same area. (Such is the case in the opening example.) It is not uncommon for one topic of debate to involve statistical issues of design and/or analysis, and it is clear from examining the medical literature that the methods of statistics are central to the vast majority of studies, a point reinforced by the following quotation:

> If for medical journals the 1960s and 1970s seem likely to be remembered as the era when the importance of ethics was emphasised, the last 10 years of this century promise to be that of statistics.
>
> *Lock (1982)*

Clinicians and others who wish to learn the basics of medical statistics are well catered for in books such as those by Colton (1974), Armitage and Berry (1987) and Altman (1991). The aim of this text is, however, somewhat different with interest centring on describing and explaining the more complex statistical techniques which are increasingly being used in medical research. Consequently it will be assumed that readers are relatively familiar with topics such as t-tests, chi-square tests, linear regression and simple analysis of variance models.
A useful way to introduce the methods which will be covered is to describe briefly a number of medical applications in which they have been used. This will be done in the next section of this opening chapter. Chapters 2–4 discuss, respectively, the design of medical investigations, the assessment of the reliability and validity of measurements, and general points about significance tests including power, sample size determination and meta-analysis. The remaining chapters discuss particular classes of technique.

1.2 Statistical methods in medical research — some examples

(a) Regression
One of the most widely used classes of statistical technique is that of *regression*, used to investigate and describe the relationship between a *dependent* variable and a number of *independent*, or *explanatory* variables. In some cases the purpose of the analysis is *prediction*, in others it is simply to discover important prognostic variables. Different types of regression method are available, corresponding to the different types of response variable that may occur in practice. Simple *linear regression* and *multiple regression*, for example, are appropriate for continuous response variables such as blood pressure or weight. *Logistic regression* is applicable to situations involving *binary* response variables, for example, 'recovered' or 'not recovered', or 'dead' or 'alive' perhaps, at the end of a treatment trial.
An interesting example of the use of linear regression for prediction is described in Bhargava *et al.* (1985). In Third World countries difficulties are often encountered in weighing newborn babies and identifying those at risk because of low birth weight. Consequently Bhargava and his co-authors searched for simpler measurements that could be substituted for weight to identify neonates with a low birth weight. A regression analysis was used to derive an equation relating measurements of mid-arm circumference, head

circumference, chest circumference and length, to bodyweight, using 520 infants born in hospital and weighed accurately. The derived equation could then be used in the field to predict birth weight from the circumference and length measurements, these being relatively easily to make even in the most difficult conditions.

Logistic regression is now widely used in medical research since many studies involve two-category response variables. An early example of the use of this technique is described in Truett *et al.* (1967) in the context of a *cohort study* (see Chapter 2) of 12-year incidence of coronary heart disease. Seven different factors measured at initial examination were studied for their effects on the incidence of the disease; they were:

(1) Age (years)
(2) Serum cholesterol (mg/dl)
(3) Systolic blood pressure (mm Hg)
(4) Relative weight
(5) Haemoglobin (g/dl)
(6) Cigarettes smoked per day
(7) ECG (normal or abnormal)

Age and cholesterol level were found to be the most important prognostic variables.

A further example of logistic regression is given in Balarajan *et al.* (1985). Here a subject's state of health, classified as chronic illness or otherwise, was related to smoking behaviour, age, sex and socioeconomic group. The main purpose of the analysis was to determine whether chronic illness was more prevalent in smokers after adjustment for age, sex and socioeconomic group.

Both types of regression are discussed in Chapter 5.

(b) Repeated Measures Analysis of Variance and Analysis of Covariance
Many medical investigations involve repeated observations of a quantitative outcome measured on every subject at several pre-defined times since the start of treatment. These *repeated measurements* over time are often accompanied by one or more pre-treatment (baseline) measurements for each subject. Commonly these studies involve several groups of subjects. The question of most interest is whether or not the different groups (frequently corresponding to different treatments), behave differently over time. To address this question it is often necessary to control for differences in the baseline measurements of the groups by a technique known as *analysis of covariance*. An example of this procedure is described by Frison and Pocock (1992). A randomized trial of 152 patients with coronary heart disease compared an active drug with a placebo during a 12-month follow-up period. The liver enzyme PK in serum was measured to study a possible adverse drug effect on the liver. Each patient had three pre-treatment measurements taken two months before, one month before and at randomization, and eight post-treatment measurements, taken every 1.5 months after randomization.

The analysis of repeated measure designs and the analysis of covariance are described in Chapter 6.

(c) Crossover Trials

A design much favoured in medical research for the comparison of two treatments is the 2×2 *crossover*. In such a design each subject receives both of two treatments, A and B. Half the subjects receive the treatments in the order AB and half in the order BA. Statistical analysis is based on within-subject comparisons and consequently allows a more precise assessment of the treatment difference. More complex crossover designs are occasionally used in the comparison of more than two treatments. An example of the use of the crossover design is given in Dennerstein *et al.* (1985) in an investigation of the use of oral micronised progesterone as a treatment for premenstrual complaints. One group of women received the progesterone for two months followed by the placebo for a further two months and a second group received the treatments in the reverse order.

Although such studies may appear at first sight to be relatively straightforward to analyse, there are, in fact, a number of potential problems. Crossover studies are also discussed in Chapter 6.

(d) Survival Analysis

In many medical investigations one of the principal variables of interest is the time until a particular event of interest occurs, for example, the time to death of a patient. Often the researcher is interested in comparing the distributions of such times in two groups of patients (treated versus not treated, for example). The comparison is usually made more difficult because of the presence of *censored* observations. Such observations involve patients for whom, by the end of the study, the event of interest has not yet occurred. In addition to comparing the *survival times* of various groups of patients, the investigator is often interested in assessing the effects of prognostic variables such as age, sex, etc., on the time variable. A suitable technique for this situation is a type of regression developed by Cox (1972). An example of the use of Cox's regression is reported by Umen and Le (1986) in an investigation of the factors associated with the survival of end-stage renal diseased patients on haemodialysis. A model for non-diabetics identified five important prognostic factors: age at initiation of dialysis, arteriosclerotic heart disease, cerebrovascular accident, cancer and chronic obstructive pulmonary disease. For diabetics, age at initiation of dialysis was the only significant prognostic variable.

A further example provided by Cook and Pocock (1987), involves the use of Cox's regression in the analysis of data from a placebo-controlled randomized clinical trial of the drug D-Penicillamine (D-P) for the treatment of primary biliary cirrhosis, a rare liver disease. Several biochemical markers in the blood, including bilirubin, albumin and aspartate transaminase, were found to have a powerful influence on patient survival.

Techniques for the analysis of survival data, including Cox's regression, are described in Chapter 7.

(e) Cluster Analysis

Classification is a fundamental process in most branches of sciences and medicine is no exception. To understand and treat disease it has to be classified and the classification will have two main aims. The first will be *prediction*, separating diseases that require different treatments. The second will be to provide a basis for research into the aetiology of diseases. Numerical methods of classification are usually referred to as techniques for *cluster analysis*, and such methods have been used in several branches of medicine. In particular, clustering has been used in psychiatry in an attempt to refine or redefine existing diagnostic categories.

An example of the use of cluster analysis for the classification of suicide attempters is provided by Paykel and Rassaby (1978). From a number of clinical studies it is evident that people who attempt suicide are very heterogeneous, spanning a range of severity of attempt, apparent motivation, previous history and other phenomena. Clearly, the treatment of such patients, and investigations of the prime causes of attempted suicide, would benefit if they could be classified in a meaningful and informative manner. With this in mind, Paykel and Rassaby studied 236 suicide attempters presenting at the main emergency service of one city in the United States. From the pool of available variables, 14 were selected as particularly relevant to classification; these included age, number of previous suicide attempts, severity of depression, severity of hostility and a rating of the overall severity of the attempt in terms of medical consequences and intention to end life. Additionally a number of demographic characteristics were recorded. Several clustering methods were applied to the 236 patients as described by the 14 chosen variables, and the final classification selected was one with three groups having the following general descriptions.

Group 1: Patients taking overdoses, on the whole showing less risk to life, less psychiatric disturbance, and more evidence of interpersonal rather than self-destructive motivation.

Group 2. Patients in this group made more serious attempts, with more self-destructive motivation and by more violent methods than overdoses.

Group 3: Patients in this group had a previous history of many attempts and gestures. Their recent attempt was relatively mild and they were overtly hostile, engendering reciprocal hostility in the psychiatrist responsible for their treatment.

The derived classification was thought likely to be extremely valuable as a basis for future studies into the causes and treatment of attempted suicide. Readers interested in other applications of cluster analysis in psychiatry are referred to Paykel (1971, 1972).

Cluster analysis is the subject of Chapter 9.

(f) Discriminant Function Analysis

An extremely important problem in many areas of medicine is that of the accurate diagnosis of a patient's complaint. By examining the patient for a number of signs or symptoms, the clinician may have to make a diagnosis which can only be positively confirmed by, say, post-mortem examination. A statistical technique which can be helpful in the area of diagnosis is *discriminant function analysis*, which begins with a sample of patients already diagnosed as having or not having a particular diseases of interest (the diagnosis having been made, for example, by a post-mortem). On each patient a set of variable values has been recorded, and a function of these variable values is derived which minimizes the number of misclassfications into disease and no disease classes for these patients. Such a function can now be applied to the variable values of *new* patients and the results used to assess whether or not they are likely to have the disease.

An example of the use of discriminant analysis is given in Allen (1983), where the technique is applied to data on acute stroke patients in order to develop an aid to diagnosis. Subsequent analyses showed that the method provided more accurate diagnoses than those provided by the treating clinician.

Discriminant function analysis is described in Chapter 11.

(g) Time Series Analysis

Many medical investigations involve long series of observations on one or more variables made at successive points in time. One example is a continuous trace from an electroencephalogram (EEG) sampled at regular intervals over some period of time. Another is monthly records of the number of cases of a particular disease taken over many years. Such a series, involving monthly notifications of chicken-pox and mumps for New York City from 1928 to 1960, is described in Helfenstein (1986), and analysed by a technique known as ARIMA or *Box–Jenkins modelling*. Such models are often useful in uncovering the mechanism that generates the time series and/or forecasting future values of the series. Helfenstein found that the number of new cases of both chicken-pox and mumps in a month is determined by the number of cases reported in the previous month plus a random component. Both series could be described by models that contained only three parameters.

ARIMA models and other methods for analysing time-series data are described in Chapter 11.

(h) Log-linear Models

Data collected in medical investigations often involve categorical variables. When such variables are cross-classified against one another a *contingency table* is formed. The analysis of such a table created from two categorical variables, involves the use of the chi-square statistic to test for independence, and will be familiar to most readers. The analysis of tables arising from three of more variables is less straightforward but is now handled routinely using *log-linear models*. An example of the use of the technique in medical research is provided by Bentley *et al.* (1983), in an investigation to assess the effects of dental health education on the use of dental health care by school children. The main analysis involved the application of log-linear analysis to the counts in a five-dimensional contingency table constructed from the variables: education, assigned dental delivery, utilization, grade and disease level.

Log-linear models and a number of other methods particularly suitable for the analysis of observational data are described in Chapter 12.

1.3 Summary

Although simple statistical techniques such as the *t*-test and chi-square test are those used most frequently by medical researchers, more complex methods such as logistic regression, survival analysis and cluster analysis are becoming increasingly important to those investigating complex medical data. It is such techniques which are the subjects of the remainder of this text.

2

The Design of Medical Investigations: Clinical Trials, Observational Studies and Surveys

2.1 Introduction

Medical investigations can be broadly classified into the *experimental* and the *observational*. The two classes are differentiated essentially by the amount of control the investigator has over what happens to the individuals being studied. In an observational study the researcher collects information but does not influence events. Groups of smokers and non-smokers may, for example, have their systolic blood pressure recorded and a test made of whether there is any evidence of a difference. The investigator does *not*, however, have the option of allocating some individuals to be smokers and others to be non-smokers. Observational studies are the foundation of *epidemiology*, the study of the causes or aetiology of diseases, and have three main aims:

(1) to describe the distribution and size of disease problems in human populations,
(2) to identify aetiological factors in the pathogenesis of disease,
(3) to provide the data essential for the management, education and planning of services for the prevention, control and treatment of disease.

By contrast, in an experimental study, the researcher can deliberately influence events and assess the effect of the intervention. The most common example involves the evaluation of a new treatment for some particular disease. Here some individuals may be given the new treatment and some the existing treatment, but which individual receives which is under the control of the investigator. (How this control is exercised is of great practical importance, and will be discussed in the next section.) Experimental studies include clinical trials and most animal laboratory studies.

2.2 Clinical trials

The aim of many medical investigations is to compare two or more treatments and to select the one that is most effective in dealing with some disease or disorder. Such investigations are not new, indeed they are as old as medicine itself — witness Bradford Hill's witch doctor trying out for the first time 'a new and nauseating compound' and comparing results with earlier and probably equally nauseating preparations (Bradford Hill, 1962). Such personal observations must have been of great importance in the advancement of medicine, particularly in its early days, and they clearly still have a role to play. Unfortunately, individual differences in the reactions of patients to diseases and therapies are often extremely variable, and personal observations on a small number of patients, however acutely and accurately made, are unlikely to tell the whole or even the appropriate story. They will often fail to agree with similar observations made by other clinicians and, as a consequence, the literature might be filled with conflicting claims and assertions. It is not unknown for this type of *ad hoc* approach to evaluating particular treatments to lead to the establishment of unjustified, or occasionally even harmful methods. Blood-letting, purging and starvation are early examples. More recently portacaval shunts for oesophageal varices and gastric freezing for duodenal ulcer, originally recommended on the basis of the results obtained from unsatisfactory and uncontrolled trials, have eventually been shown to do more harm than good.

Clearly then, there is a need for some form of adequately controlled procedure to assess the advantages and disadvantages of different treatments. Such a need has become even more acute over the last two decades or so with the ever increasing production of new drugs. The need has largely been met by the wide use and general acceptance of the *controlled clinical trial*, the case for which was clearly put as long ago as 1949, by Pickering, in his Presidential address to the Section of Experimental Medicine and Therapeutics of the Royal Society of Medicine.

Therapeutics is the branch of medicine that, by its very nature, should be experimental. For if we take a patient affected with a malady, and we alter his conditions of life, either by dieting him, or putting him to bed, or by administering to him a drug, or by performing on him an operation, we are performing an experiment. And if we are scientifically minded we should record the results. Before concluding that the change for better or for worse in the patient is due to the specific treatment employed, we must ascertain whether the result can be repeated a significant number of times in similar patients, whether the result was merely due to the natural history of the disease, or in other words to the lapse of time, or whether it was due to some other factor which was necessarily associated with the therapeutic measure in question. And if, as a result of these procedures, we learn that the therapeutic measure employed produces a significant, though not very pronounced improvement, we would experiment with the method, altering dosage or other detail to see if it can be improved. This would seem the procedure to be expected of men with six years of scientific training behind them. But it has not been followed. Had it been done we should have gained a fairly precise knowledge of the place of individual methods of therapy in disease, and our efficiency as doctors would have been enormously enhanced.

Pickering (1949)

A case which amply illustrates Pickering's concern is that involving penicillin. Alexander Fleming noticed the antibacterial effect of the mould *Penicillium notatum* in the early 1930s but failed to study these effects systematically. It was not until a decade later that two researchers, having happened upon Fleming's original paper, injected the compound into four sick mice whilst leaving another four untreated and crossed the boundary from anecdote to scientific evidence. (Nevertheless Fleming was regarded as a hero and awarded the Nobel Prize!)

Clinical trials have, over the 40 years since Pickering's address, become of paramount importance in investigations of new drugs and other treatments. As pointed out by Bradford Hill (1962), however, they are, in essence at least, far from new, and it is well worthwhile spending a moment considering an 18th century study described by Lind (1753), since it illustrates a number of features still relevant to today's trials. The following quotation from Lind's account is given by Bradford Hill.

On the 20th May, 1747, I took twelve patients in the scurvy, on board the *Salisbury* at sea. Their cases were as similar as I could have them. They all in general had putrid gums, the spots and lassitude, with weakness of their knees. They lay together in one place, being a proper apartment for the sick in the fore-hold; and had one diet in common to all, viz. water-gruel sweetned with sugar in the morning; fresh mutton broth often times for dinner; at other times puddings, boiled biscuit with sugar etc. And for supper, barley and raisins, rice and currants, sago and wine, or the like. Two of these were ordered each a quart of cider a day. Two others took twenty-five gutts of *elixir vitriol* three times a day, upon an empty stomach; using a gargle strongly acidulated with it for their mouths. Two others took two spoonfuls of vinegar three times a day, upon an empty stomach; having their gruels and their other food well acidulated with it, as also the gargle for their mouths. Two of the worst patients, with the tendons in the ham rigid (a symptom none of the rest had) were put under a course of sea-water. Of this they drank half a pint every day, and sometimes more or less as it operated, by way of a gentle physic. Two others had each two oranges and one lemon given them every day. These they eat with greediness, at different times, upon an empty stomach. They continued but six days under this course, having consumed the quantity that could be spared. The two remaining patients, took the bigness of a nutmeg three times a day of an electuary recommended by a hospital-surgeon, made of garlic, mustard-feed, *rad.raphan*, balsam of *Peru*, and gum myrr; using for common drink barley water well acidulated with tamarinds; by a decoction of which, with the addition of *cremor tartar*, they were greatly purged three or four times during the course.

The consequence was, that the most sudden and visible good effects were perceived from the use of the oranges and lemons; one of those who had taken them, being at the end of six days fit for duty. The spots were not indeed at that time quite off his body, nor his gums sound; but without any other medicine, than a gargle of *elixir vitriol*, he became quite healthy before we came into Plymouth, which was on the 16th June. The other was the best recovered of any in his condition; and being now deemed pretty well, was appointed nurse to the rest of the sick.

Lind's experiment illustrates two essential features of a clinical trial; firstly, it involves *comparison* — a group of individuals submitted to a new treatment is compared with a group given the old treatment. (Both might be compared with a group given a placebo in a modern trial.) Secondly, Lind had some method for assessing the *outcome* of the trial. It is not altogether clear how Lind decided which individuals should receive which treatment, but in today's controlled clinical trial, the most usual, and in general the most satisfactory, procedure for deciding this is *random allocation*. Whether a patient receives the new or old treatment (or perhaps a placebo), is decided, for example, by the toss of a coin, or by some other convenient random procedure.

2.2.1 Randomization and medical ethics

Random allocation gives all subjects the same chance of receiving either treatment. Randomization serves several purposes; it provides an important method of allocating treatments to patients free from personal biases, and it ensures a firm basis for the application of significance tests and most of the rest of the statistical methodology likely to be used in assessing the results of the trial. Most importantly randomization distributes the effects of concomitant variables, both measured and unobserved (and possibly unknown), in a chance, and therefore impartial, fashion amongst the groups to be compared. In these ways, random allocation ensures a lack of bias, making the interpretation of an observed group difference largely unambiguous — its cause is very likely the different treatments or conditions received by the different groups.

Randomized controlled trials are now widely used in medical research. Recent examples include a trial of psychotherapy for bulimia nervosa (Freeman *et al.* 1988) and one for low dose β blockers in acute stroke (Barer *et al.* 1988). Unfortunately, however, the idea that patients should be randomly assigned to treatments is not appealing to many clinicians nor to many of the prospective participants in a trial. Reasons for their concern are not difficult to identify. The clinician faced with the responsibility of restoring the patient to health and suspecting that any new treatment is likely to have advantages over the old, may be unhappy that many patients will be receiving, in her view, the less valuable treatment. The patient being recruited for a trial, having been made aware of the randomization component, might be troubled by the possibility of receiving an 'inferior' treatment.

Because of such worries, alternatives to random allocation are sometimes considered. The most common is to allow all suitable patients to receive the new treatment and to compare their responses and outcomes with those obtained from the records of patients previously given the old treatment, the so called *historical controls*. The use of such a control group makes the considerable assumption that everything, except the new treatment under test, has remained constant in time. So, for example, the type of patient, the severity of the illness the ancillary treatment given and the measurements made must all be the same for any observed difference in response to be attributed to the different treatments received. It is only rarely that an investigator can risk giving much credence to this assumption. Past observations are unlikely to relate to a precisely similar group of patients, the quality of information extracted from the historical controls is likely to be different (probably inferior) since such patients were not initially intended to be part of the trial. Patients given a new, and yet unproven, treatment are likely to be far more closely monitored and receive more intensive care than historical controls receiving the orthodox treatment in a routine manner.

Table 2.1 Published clinical trials for six medical issues (taken with permission from Sacks *et al.*, 1983).

	Randomized trials		Historical control trials	
Therapy	*New treatment effective*	*New treatment ineffective*	*New treatment effective*	*New treatment ineffective*
Coronary artery surgery	1	7	16	5
Anticoagulants for acute myocardial infarction	1	9	5	1
Surgery for oesophaeal varices	0	8	4	1
Fluorouracil (5-FU) for colon cancer	0	5	2	0
BCG immunotherapy for melanoma	2	2	4	0
Diethylstilbesterol for habitual abortion	0	3	5	0

For these, and a variety of other reasons (see Pocock, 1983), studies with historical controls are very likely to *overestimate* the efficacy of a new treatment. Apart from the obvious disadvantages of such exaggerated claims, they also make it more difficult to arrange properly randomized trials since many clinicians may be reluctant to randomize patients to a treatment that they consider from previous evidence (i.e. the historical controls study), to be inferior. Some evidence for the possible bias produced by the use of historical control trials is provided by Sacks *et al.* (1983), who compare the inferences of published trials in similar areas, some of which involved randomisation and others the use of historical controls. The results are shown in Table 2.1. The historical control studies show a preponderance of results in favour of the new treatment. (Some arguments in favour of the use of historical controls in specific circumstances are made in Gehan and Freireich, 1974 and in Gehan, 1983. In particular, when the number of patients available for a randomized controlled trial is limited, the case for considering using historical controls is strengthened, a point taken up in detail by Pocock, 1976.)

Randomized controlled clinical trials are now widely considered to be the most scientifically valid method of evaluating the risks and benefits of medical innovations. Even in a properly randomized controlled trial however, the comparison of treatments may still be distorted if the patient and/or the physician responsible for treatment and evaluation of outcome, know which treatment the patient is receiving. Such a problem is avoided by the *double-blind* trial in which neither patient nor clinician is aware of which treatment the patient is receiving. In the case of oral drug therapy, the double-blind approach is usually relatively straightforward to implement, since it is generally easy to manufacture an oral placebo which is identical in all respects to the active therapy except of course, in not possessing the active ingredient. Double-blind studies in other situations (those involving surgery or repeated injections, for example), are much less easy and often impossible to arrange although an interesting and unusual example involving electroconvulsive therapy is described in Johnstone *et al.* (1980). In such cases potential biases in treatment comparisons can be lessened, or even removed entirely, by arranging for assessment and evaluation of outcome to be carried out blind, the assessor not knowing the treatment the patient received.

But despite the wide acceptance of the randomized controlled trial there is still concern amongst many clinicians that such trials can violate the doctor–patient relationship. The ethical problem involves the conflict between trying to ensure that each individual patient receives the treatment most beneficial for his condition, and evaluating competing therapies as efficiently as possible so that all future patients might benefit from the superior treatment. Lellouch and Schwartz (1971) refer to the problem as competition between *individual* and *collective* ethics. Pocock (1983) suggests that each clinical trial requires a balance between the two. The prime motivation for conducting a trial involves collective ethics, but individual ethics have to be given as much attention as possible without destroying the trial's validity. A very important point made by Pocock is that it is unethical to conduct trials which are of sufficiently poor quality that they cannot make a meaningful contribution to medical knowledge.

Such points have a number of implications for clinicians considering taking part in a randomized controlled trial, which are nicely summarized in the following two quotations.

(1) Patients should not be admitted who could not be assigned without hesitation to any of the study therapies by all of the participating physicians. For one physician to admit patients that another would reject is ethically inappropriate and scientifically undesirable.

(2) Assume that several physicians believe that a scientific clinical trial is needed and is ethical ... what should the physician who rather reluctantly agrees that *perhaps* a trial is desirable do? Such a physician should stay out of the study unless he can faithfully and in good conscience follow without bias the specific rules of the study. A physician's behaviour is both unethical and unscientific if he joins a study and then begins to undermine its soundness by biased actions.

Shaw and Chalmers (1970)

Naturally the physician's responsibilities to patients during the course of a trial are clear; if the patient's condition deteriorates, the ethical obligation must always and entirely outweigh any experimental conditions. This obligation means that whenever a physician thinks that the interests of her patients are at stake, she must be allowed to treat the patient as she sees fit. This is an absolutely essential requirement for an ethically conducted trial, no matter what complications it may introduce into the final analyses of the data.

A further reason why the statistician and the clinician involved in a randomized controlled clinical trial may come into conflict concerns the decision when to call a halt to the trial. This is a possibility since, as results came in, they may

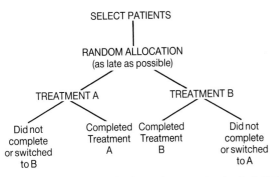

Figure 2.1 A simplified schema for a randomized clinical trial (reproduced with permission from Newell, 1992).

appear to indicate the superiority of one treatment over another. If they do the clinician may be inclined to ask for the trial to be stopped in order to avoid some patients continuing to receive the 'inferior' treatment. The statistician may argue, however, that the perceived difference between the treatments is illusory and ask for the trial to run its course for the time originally intended. Such possible conflict raises important, and often difficult, statistical as well as ethical issues that are taken up in detail in Chapter 4.

The analysis of data arising from randomized clinical trials usually involves, at least in the initial stages, relatively straightforward application of standard statistical tests such as the *t*-test, etc. A complication that arises in many trials is that of patients who fail to complete the intended course of treatment, and who are either removed from the trial or in some cases switched to the alternative therapy group or a therapy different from any prescribed in the protocol. Figure 2.1 shows a diagrammatic representation of the possibilities.

Statistically the appropriate way of dealing with the observations arising from such a trial is by *intention-to-treat* analysis. Essentially this means that all patients randomly allocated to one of the treatments in a trial should be analysed together as representing that treatment, whether or not they completed, or even received that treatment. In intention-to-treat analysis, the randomization not only decides the allocated treatment, it decides there and then how the patient's data will be analysed, whether or not the patient actually receives the prescribed treatment.

Analysis based on intention-to-treat may appear to offend intuition and clinicians may often press for comparisons based on the treatment actually received rather than the treatment prescribed. There are however several arguments against this approach. First, the prognostic balance brought about by randomization is likely to be disturbed and so the validity of the statistical test procedures will be undermined. Second, results of analysis by treatment received may suffer from a bias introduced by using compliance, a factor often related to outcome, to determine the groups for comparison.

Excellent accounts of the intention-to-treat principle which include a number of examples of what can go wrong if the principle is not implemented, are given in Newell (1992) and Peduzzi *et al.* (1991).

The randomized double-blind controlled trial is the 'gold-standard' against which to judge the quality of clinical trials in general. But such trials are still misunderstood by many clinicians, and questions about whether or not they are ethical persist (Burkhardt and Kienle, 1978). One of the problems, identified by Bracken (1987), is that doctors are frequently reluctant to accept their uncertainty about much of what they practise. Bracken concludes that when doctors *are* able to admit to themselves and their patients uncertainty about the best action, then no conflict exists between the roles of the doctor and the scientist. In such circumstances it cannot be less ethical to choose a treatment by random allocation within a controlled trial than to choose by what happens to be readily available, hunch, or what a drug company recommends. The most effective argument in favour of randomized clinical trials is that the alternative, practising in complacent uncertainty, is worse.

(Many more details of the ethical and methodological issues in clinical trials are discussed in a series of papers in a special issue of *Statistics in Medicine*—Volume 12, 1993.)

2.3 Surveys and observational studies

Much of medical research is concerned with the investigation of the relationship between possible risk factors and the development of a particular disease or condition. Recent examples include those of passive smoking and lung cancer (Hole *et al.,* 1989), caffeine consumption in pregnant women and infant birthweight (Brooke *et al.,* 1989) and job loss and health (Iversen *et al.,* 1989). There is no logical difference between comparing the outcome of two groups of patients receiving different exposures to a risk factor and two groups of patients given alternative treatments. But in areas of epidemiological research such as the former, random allocation of patients to groups is not a possibility, and the researcher must rely on an observational study to provide evidence of a relationship or *association* between the risk factor and the disease. In such studies the exposure to the risk factor may have been self-imposed (for example, smoking) or it may have arisen because of geographical location (for example, an atmospheric pollutant) or occupation (for example, exposure to asbestos).

Evidence that a suspected risk factor is associated with a particular disease may be obtained in a variety of ways. Early investigations may simply involve the study of vital statistics such as those provided in government publications. A fascinating example is provided by Alderson (1983) who describes the events surrounding the dense fog suffered in London during the four days 5–8 December, 1952. Figure 2.2 shows a plot of total deaths and air pollution levels measured during the period of the fog. The graph is very suggestive of a link between the level of atmospheric pollution and number of daily deaths recorded during the fog.

Examination of mortality and morbidity statistics frequently provides the first clue to possible associations of interest. The next stage often involves some form of *survey* which collects information from individuals about their history, habits, knowledge, attitudes or behaviour. A recent example is a survey seeking information on knowledge about AIDS (Bellingham and Gillies, 1993). A readable account of designing surveys is given in Alderson (1983).

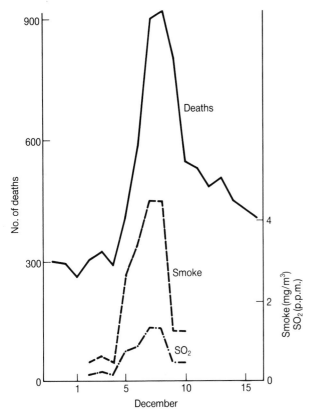

Figure 2.2 Total deaths in Greater London and air pollution levels measured during the fog of December 1952 (reproduced with permission from Alderson, 1983).

The three main types of observational investigation are the *cohort* or *prospective* study, the *retrospective* or *case-control* study, and the *cross-sectional* study, each of which will now be discussed in detail. Figure 2.3 illustrates the basic difference between the three procedures.

2.3.1 Prospective studies

Prospective studies begin with the identification of two groups of people, the members of one group having been exposed to the risk factor, and those in the other group not having been exposed. The people in each group are then followed forward in time to determine what happens to them with respect to the illness under investigation. Figure 2.4 illustrates the process diagrammatically.

A classic example of a prospective study is that undertaken by Hill and Doll in the 1950s (Doll and Hill, 1954) to investigate the possible link between smoking and the development of lung cancer. In 1951 they wrote to all practitioners on the medical register in the United Kingdom and included a brief self-completion questionnaire about smoking habits. This material was then collated with subsequent information on the mortality of the respondents.

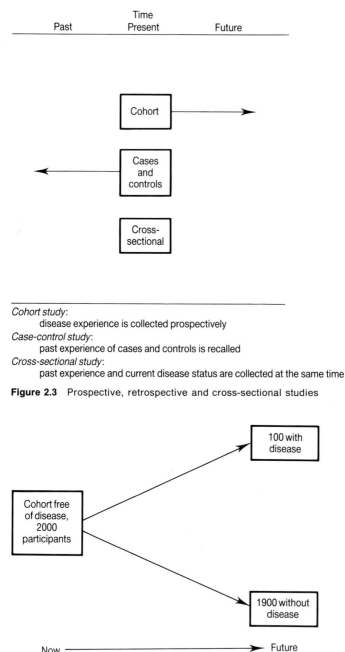

Cohort study:
    disease experience is collected prospectively
Case-control study:
    past experience of cases and controls is recalled
Cross-sectional study:
    past experience and current disease status are collected at the same time

Figure 2.3   Prospective, retrospective and cross-sectional studies

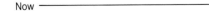

Figure 2.4   Prospective study

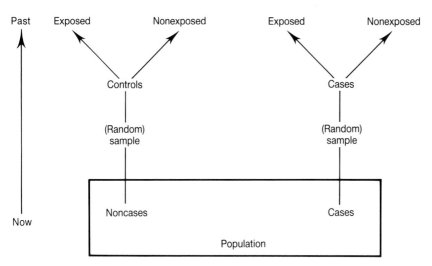

Figure 2.5 Retrospective study

More recent examples include an investigation of factors associated with childhood cancer, reported in Golding *et al.* (1990) and a study of birthweight and length of gestation in a population surrounding a lead smelter—Litvak *et al.* (1991).

A prospective study resembles the experimental approach of the controlled clinical trial, although an observed difference in the incidence of the disease in the two groups, at the end of a specified time period, cannot unambiguously be attributed to the risk factor because of the lack of random allocation. Nevertheless, this type of study does provide a more direct test of a specific hypothesis on aetiology than the rival, case-control, approach (see next section). The main disadvantage of the prospective study is that can take a long time and may be very expensive. In the case of very rare diseases a large number of people would be needed at the outset to ensure that comparisons of incident rates at the end of the study were based on reasonable numbers. A further disadvantage is that of patients who 'fall by the wayside'. Such patients may introduce bias into any analysis because of differences from those patients who remain in the study. Alderson (1983) gives some examples.

2.3.2 Case-control studies

The case-control study begins with the identification of a group of subjects with the disease or condition of interest (the cases) and an unaffected group (the controls). Then for each case and each control the investigator collects information about their past history in an attempt to assess their past exposure to the risk factor of interest. Figure 2.5 illustrates the case-control study diagrammatically.

One example of a case-control study was that conducted in a number of hospitals in several large American cities to investigate the possible link between the use of oral contraceptives and thromboembolic disease. During a three-year period, all married women from age 15 to 44 who were discharged from these hospitals with a diagnosis of idiopathic thromboembolism (blood clots) were identified. For each identified case, a control was selected. Controls were female patients discharged alive from the same hospitals in the same six-month time period; additionally they were individually matched to the thomboembolism cases on age, marital status, race, etc. The history of each woman's oral contraceptive usage was investigated in a series of interviews.

A further example of a case-control study is described in Neugut *et al.* (1989), whose interest was in investigating a possible inverse relationship between serum cholesterol level and risk of cancer, particularly primary brain tumours. Cases consisted of patients registered in the Columbia Presbyterian Medical Center Tumor Registry with a diagnosis of primary brain tumour between 1 January 1980 and 31 December 1983 and over the age of 45. Controls consisted of patients with three diagnoses: herniorrhaphy, herniated lumbar disc disease and prolapsed uterus. These patients were selected as controls because their conditions have no known or suspected association with serum cholesterol level, and they were admitted to the hospital on an elective or semi-elective basis, similar to the group of cases.

The main advantages of the retrospective, case-control study over prospective investigations are that they require considerably shorter study time, are relatively inexpensive and more suitable for examining links with rare diseases. They do however also suffer from a number of considerable disadvantages. Firstly selection of an appropriate control group is not always straightforward. Ideally, the controls should be as similar as possible to the cases, except that they do not have the condition being investigated. But often, subjects who do not have the outcome of interest may well differ in other ways from the cases; in particular they may be atypical with regard to the exposure of interest. A method frequently used to ensure that cases and controls are comparable is to match on variables such as sex, age, occupation, etc., that might possibly confound any comparison. Selecting controls for this type of study is discussed in detail in Alderson (1983).

A second possible problem with the case-control study is the manner in which information regarding the presence or absence of the risk factor is derived. Suppose, for example, the required information is to be collected from previous records. It is easy to see that this might often lead to spuriously observing a higher frequency of the risk factor amongst the cases rather than the controls, simply because, when the records were being made, the risk factor was looked for more closely in the cases than in the controls. In the latter group mention of the risk factor might be excluded from the record merely because the relevant question was not deemed to be of interest and therefore was not asked. Eliciting the information required in a retrospective study by means of personal interviews with both cases and controls might be seen as a way of overcoming the obvious problems with using previous records, and in many cases is likely to provide a more valid comparison. The possibility remains, however, of extracting different responses in the two groups. Vessey and Doll (1969), for example, suggest that in studies investigating oral contraceptives as a possible risk factor for particular diseases, a woman's ability and willingness to recall details of her contraceptive history may be affected by whether she has suffered an illness which might be associated in her mind with the type of contraceptive she had used.

It is not unknown for prospective and retrospective studies of the same area to come to different conclusions. In investigations of the possible link between the use of X-rays on pregnant women and the development of acute leukaemia in their children, for example, both prospective and retrospective approaches have been used. In the latter, 10% of mothers of children developing the disease had undergone diagnostic X-rays whilst pregnant and about 5% of control mothers (of healthy control children), had been so X-rayed. In the prospective study, all pregnant mothers irradiated in a few large hospitals were considered and the medical history of their children observed for several years. The incidence of leukaemia was found to be slightly *below* the national average, in contradiction to the finding from the retrospective study.

Several explanations are possible both for the large difference found in the retrospective investigation and for the difference between the results in the two types of study. Rather than believing that the use of X-rays doubles the risk of leukaemia to the child (as suggested by the figures from the retrospective study taken at their face value), for example, it might be argued that the mothers were X-rayed *because* a problem with their pregnancy was suspected, and the mothers with leukaemic children were the ones more likely to have some symptoms and thus be X-rayed.

Other possible explanations for the different findings from the prospective and retrospective study are:

(1)   there were inevitable biases in the retrospective study,
(2)   the numbers in the prospective study were too small,
(3)   combined with (2), the particular 'large' hospital used had 'safer' X-ray apparatus than most others.

2.3.3 The Cross-sectional study

The cross-sectional survey is distinct from the prospective and retrospective studies described above since it does not involve the passing of time. This type of study simply provides a 'snapshot' view of an area. Most surveys provide information of this type. Rasmussen and Olesen (1992), for example, examined the relationship between headaches and psychosocial factors by asking 1000 people to complete a detailed questionnaire, and Römelsjö (1989) investigated the association between alcohol consumption and social status in Stockholm by using a postal questionnaire followed-up by a telephone interview.

In all types of observational study, conclusions about possible *causal* links between risk factors and disease are hard to make, this being particularly true for the cross-sectional study. In such a study concerned with the possible link between smoking and high blood pressure, for example, suppose a higher incidence of high blood pressure is found amongst the smokers. Possible explanations for the observed association are:

(1)   smoking causes an increase in blood pressure,
(2)   people with high blood pressure tend to smoke more,

(3) some unidentified factor affects both the tendency to smoke and the tendency to increased blood pressure.

Methods particularly relevant for the analysis of observational studies are described in Chapter 12.

2.4 Summary

In this chapter a number of possible designs for medical investigations have been described. The controlled clinical trial, with random allocation of patients to treatment groups, is the preferred approach in those situations where it can be applied without insurmountable ethical objections, since such an experimental approach has many advantages. Indeed according to Sinclair (1951):

> the use of the experimental method has brilliant discoveries to its credit, whereas the method of observation has achieved little.

But in many cases when dealing with human subjects, such experimental studies are impossible to undertake and so observational investigations become necessary. Prospective studies are closest to the experimental approach of the clinical trial and often lead to less ambiguous conclusions than retrospective or cross-sectional methods. The researcher undertaking any type of observational investigation might do well to heed the words of Bradford Hill:

> The observer may well have to be more patient than the experimenter awaiting the occurrence of the natural succession of events he desires to study; he may have to be more imaginative — sensing the correlations that lie below the surface of his observations; and he may well have to be more logical and less dogmatic — avoiding as the evil eye the fallacy of *post hoc ergo propter hoc*, the mistaking of correlation for causation.
>
> *Bradford Hill (1962)*

More detailed descriptions of clinical trials and observational studies can be found in Pocock (1983), Alderson (1983) and in the special issue of *Statistics in Medicine* (**3** (4), 1984), devoted to the evaluation of therapy.

3

Measurement in Medicine

3.1 Introduction

> Stone-dead has no fellow, and pre-eminent, therefore, stands the number of patients who die. No statistician, so far as I know, has in this respect accused the physician of an over-reliance upon the clinical impression
>
> *Bradford Hill (1962)*

The basic material which is the foundation of all medical investigations consists of the measurements and observations which are made on the patients or subjects of interest. Clearly such measurements need to be objective, precise and reproducible for reasons nicely summarized by the following quotation from Fleiss (1986).

> The most elegant design of a clinical study will not overcome the damage caused by unreliable or imprecise measurement. The requirement that one's data be of high quality is at least as important a component of a proper study design as the requirement for randomization, double blinding, controlling where necessary for prognostic factors, and so on. Larger sample sizes than otherwise necessary, biased estimates, and even biased samples are some of the untoward consequences of unreliable measurements that can be demonstrated.

As Bradford Hill points out in the quotation which began this chapter, the death of a patient is the most objective outcome observation that might be made in a study. Fortunately, however, most trials are concerned with diseases which are not lethal, and where assessment of outcome depends on something less drastic than dead or alive at the end of the study. The appropriate measurements and observations that need to be made depend on the particular area of investigation. They may involve, for example, measurements of blood pressure, weight, temperature, etc., or ratings of anxiety, depression or degree of pain, or simply a statement of improved or not improved in respect of some course of treatment. The characteristics of the observations and measurements made will, in part at least, help to determine the appropriate methods of

Table 3.1   Classification of 141 patients
by type of cerebral tumour

(A)	Benignant tumours	78
(B)	Malignant tumours	37
(C)	Other cerebral tumours	26
		141

statistical analysis, and in the next section a general account of measurement scales is undertaken.

Requirements common to all studies in terms of measurements are, firstly, that the decision about which measurements are to be made needs to be taken *before* the trial commences. The alternative is potential chaos. Secondly, attention needs to be given to training clinicians and others on the measuring instruments to be used. This is particularly important in multi-centre studies. Lastly an assessment of inter-observer agreement and reliability on the measures needs to be made before the trial begins, particularly with measures such as psychiatric rating scales, which are likely to be less objective than say measurements of height and weight. The assessment of reliability and agreement is discussed in Section 3.3.

3.2 Scales of measurement

Clearly not all measurement is the same. Measuring an individual's weight is qualitatively different from measuring their response to some treatment on a two category scale, 'improved', 'not improved'. Measurement scales are differentiated according to the degree of precision involved. If it is said that an individual has a high serum uric acid level, it is not as precise as the statement that the individual has 8.5 mg/100mm of serum uric acid. The comment that a woman is tall is not as accurate as specifying that her height is 1.88m. Certain characteristics of interest are more amenable to precise measurement than others. Given an accurate thermometer, a patient's temperature can be measured very precisely. Quantifying the level of anxiety or depression of a psychiatric patient, or assessing the degree of pain of a migraine sufferer are, however, far more difficult tasks. Measurement scales may be classified into a hierarchy ranging from *categorical*, though *ordinal*, to *interval* and finally *ratio* scales. Each of these will now be considered in more detail.

3.2.1 Nominal or categorical data

Nominal or categorical measurements allow patients to be classified with respect to some characteristic. Table 3.1, for example, shows a classification of 141 patients by type of cerebral tumour, and Table 3.2 the classification of 5375 deaths from tuberculosis by the form of disease causing death.

Such data often become of more interest when *pairs* of categorical variables are *cross-classified* to form a *contingency table*. Table 3.3 and 3.4 are two

Table 3.2 Deaths from tuberculosis

(A)	Tuberculosis of respiratory system	4853
(B)	Other forms of tuberculosis	522
		5375

Table 3.3 Classification of 141 patients by type and site of cerebral tumour

Site	*Type* A	*B*	*C*	*Row totals*
Frontal lobes	23	9	6	38
Temporal lobes	21	4	3	28
Other cerebral areas	34	24	17	75
	78	37	26	141

examples of such tables. Contingency tables often summarize the results of an observational study and their analysis is discussed in Chapter 12.

The properties of a nominal scale are:

(1) data categories are mutually exclusive (an individual can belong to only one category),
(2) data categories have no logical order — numbers may be assigned to categories but merely as convenient labels.

A nominal scale classifies without the categories being ordered.

3.2.2 Ordinal scales

The next level in the measurement hierearchy is the *ordinal* scale. This has one additional property over those of a nominal scale — a logical ordering of the categories. With such measurements the numbers assigned to the categories indicate the amount of a characteristic possessed. A psychiatrist may, for example, grade patients on an anxiety scale as 'not anxious,' 'mildly

Table 3.4 Deaths from tuberculosis by type and sex

	Type A	*B*	*Row totals*
Male	3534	270	3804
Female	1319	252	1571
	4853	522	5375

anxious', 'moderately anxious' or 'severely anxious', and use the numbers 0, 1, 2 and 3 to label the categories, with lower numbers indicating less anxiety. The psychiatrist cannot however infer, that the *difference* in anxiety between patients with scores of say, 0 and 1, is the same as that between patients assigned scores, 2 and 3. The scores on an ordinal scale allow patients to be *ranked* with respect to the characteristic being assessed. Frequently, however, measurements on an ordinal scale are described in terms of their mean and standard deviation. This is *not* appropriate if the steps on the scale are not known to be of equal length. Andersen (1990), Chapter 15, gives a nice illustration of why this is so.

The following are the properties of an ordinal scale:

(1)   data categories are mutually exclusive,
(2)   data categories have some logical order,
(3)   data categories are scaled according to the amount of a particular characteristic they possess.

3.2.3 Interval scales

The third level in the measurement scale hierarchy is the *interval* scale. Such scales possess all the properties of an ordinal scale, plus the additional property that equal differences between category levels, on any part of the scale, reflect equal differences in the characteristic measured. An example of such a scale is temperature on the Celsius or Fahrenheit scale; the difference between temperatures of 80°F and 90°F is the same as between temperatures of 30°F and 40°F. An important point to make about interval scales is that the zero point is simply another point on the scale; it does *not* represent the starting point of the scale, nor the total absence of the characteristic being measured. The properties of an interval scale are as follows:

(1)   data categories are mutually exclusive,
(2)   data categories have a logical order,
(3)   data categories are scaled according to the amount of the characteristic they possess,
(4)   equal differences in the characteristic are represented by equal differences in the numbers assigned to the categories,
(5)   the zero point is completely arbitrary.

3.2.4 Ratio scales

The highest level in the hierarchy of measurement scales is the ratio scale. This type of scale has one property in addition to those listed for interval scales, namely the possession of a true zero point which represents the absence of the characteristic being measured. Consequently statements can be made both about differences on the scale *and* the ratio of points on the scale. An example is weight, where not only is the difference between 100 kg and 50 kg the same as between 75kg and 25kg, but an object weighing 100kg can be said to be twice as heavy as one weighing 50kg. This is not true of say temperature on the Celsius or Fahrenheit scales, where a reading of 100° does *not* represent twice the warmth of a temperature of 50°. If, however, the temperatures were measured on the Kelvin scale, which does have a true zero point, the statement about the ratio could be made.

The properties of a ratio scale are:

(1) data categories are mutually exclusive,
(2) data categories have a logical order,
(3) data categories are scaled according to the amount of the characteristic they possess,
(4) equal differences in the characteristic are represented by equal differences in the numbers assigned to the categories,
(5) the zero point represents an absence of the characteristic being measured.

3.3 Observer bias, reliability and validity

In all studies it is important to be sure that the data collected are as accurate as possible. In assessing the accuracy of any particular measuring 'instrument', it is usual to distinguish between the *reliability* of the data collected and their *validity*. Reliability is essentially the extent of the agreement between repeated measurements, and validity is the extent to which a method of measurement provides a true assessment of that which it purports to measure. There are several comprehensive accounts of reliability and the statistical evaluation of measurement errors, see for example Fleiss (1986) and Dunn (1989). Here only a brief account of the area is given primarily via some numerical examples. The next section deals with measures of reliability and agreement for categorical data and Section 3.3.2 considers the same topics for data on an interval scale.

3.3.1 Reliability measures for categorical data

Fleiss (1965) and Landis and Koch (1977) suggest that when studying the variability of observer ratings, two components of possible lack of accuracy must be distinguished. The first is *inter-observer bias*, which is reflected in differences in the marginal distributions of the response variable for each of the observers. The second is *observer disagreement*, which is indicated by how observers classify individual subjects into the same category on the measurement scale.

As an illustration of the assessment of inter-observer bias consider the data shown in Table 3.5, collected during a study comparing the symptomatology of eight schizophrenic patients as judged by five psychiatrists during a psychiatric interview. The symptom involved in Table 3.5 is *religious preoccupation* rated 0 if thought to be absent and 1 if considered present. The proportion of patients rated to have the symptom present appears to differ considerably amongst the five raters. Such differences might be due simply to chance effects, however, and a more formal test of the hypothesis of no inter-observer bias is what is really required. Fleiss (1965) shows that the appropriate test for this hypothesis is *Cochran's Q-test*, the relevant test statistic being

$$Q = \frac{r(r-1)\sum_{j=1}^{r}(y_{.j} - y_{..}/r)^2}{ry_{..} - \sum_{i=1}^{n} y_{i.}^2} \tag{3.1}$$

Table 3.5   Symptomatology ratings of five psychiatrists

	Psychiatrist 1	2	3	4	5	Total	Proportion
1	0	0	0	0	0	0	0.0
2	0	0	0	0	1	1	0.2
3	0	0	0	0	0	0	0.0
4	0	0	0	0	0	0	0.0
5	0	0	1	0	0	1	0.2
6	0	0	1	1	1	3	0.6
7	0	0	0	0	0	0	0.0
8	1	0	1	1	1	4	0.8
Total	1	0	3	2	3	9	0.225
Proportion	0.125	0.000	0.375	0.250	0.375		

where n is the number of subjects, r the number of raters and
$y_{ij} = 1$ if the ith patient is judged by the jth psychiatrist to have the symptom present,
$= 0$ otherwise,
$y_{i.} =$ total number of psychiatrists who judge the ith patient to have the symptom present,
$y_{.j} =$ total number of patients the jth psychiatrist judges as having the symptoms present,
$y_{..} =$ total number of 'present' judgements made.

If the hypothesis of no inter-observer bias is true, Q has, approximately, a chi-square distribution with $r - 1$ degrees of freedom. For the data given in Table 3.5, the test statistic is calculated as

$$Q = \frac{5 \times 4 \times [(1-1.8)^2 + (0-1.8)^2 + (3-1.8)^2 + (2-1.8)^2 + (3-1.8)^2]}{45.0 - 27.0} = 7.55 \quad (3.2)$$

The associated p value found from a chi-square distribution with 4 d.f. is 0.109. The data give no evidence of inter-observer bias amongst these five psychiatrists on the particular symptom being assessed.

Of more relevance in most circumstances than inter-observer bias, is the assessment of observer agreement or reliability. One of the most common approaches to the problem for categorical data is the use of the *kappa coefficient*. To illustrate the calculation of this measure, the data shown in Table 3.6 will be used. These are part of a data set collected by Holmquist *et al.* (1967) in an investigation into observer reliability in the histological classification of carcinoma *in situ* and related lesions of the uterine cervix. In the original study seven pathologists separately classified 118 biopsy slides into one of the following five categories based on the most involved lesion:

Category 1: negative,
Category 2: atypical squamous hyperplasia,
Category 3: carcinoma *in situ*,
Category 4: squamous carcinoma with early stromal invasion,
Category 5: invasive carcinoma.

Table 3.6 Observed frequencies of biopsy slides classified by two pathologists according to most involved lesion of the uterine cervix

		Pathologist 2					
		1	2	3	4	5	Row totals
	1	22	2	2	0	0	26
	2	5	7	14	0	0	26
Pathologist 1	3	0	2	36	0	0	38
	4	0	1	14	7	0	22
	5	0	0	3	0	3	6
		27	12	69	7	3	118

Table 3.6 shows the data from just two of the pathologists.

One intuitively reasonable index of agreement for the two raters is the proportion of patients they classify into the same category; this proportion, P_0 is given by

$$P_0 = (22 + 7 + 36 + 7 + 3)/118 = 0.64 \qquad (3.3)$$

Such a measure has the virtue of simplicity. Additionally it is readily understood. Nevertheless it is not an adequate index, since it ignores agreement between the raters that might be due to chance. To illustrate this problem consider Tables 3.7 and 3.8. In both, the two observers are measured as achieving 66% agreement using P_0 in (3.2). Suppose, however, that each observer was simply allocating patients at random to the diagnostic categories in accordance with their marginal rates. Observer 1 of Table 3.7 would, for example, simply allocate 10% of patients to category 1, 40% to category 2 and the remaining 10% to category 3, without regard to the actual condition of the patients involved. Such a procedure would lead to some agreement between the two observers, resulting in a non-zero value of P_0. This *chance* agreement, P_c, can be calculated simply from the marginal rates of each observer. In Table 3.7 it is given by

$$P_c = \frac{1}{100}\left[\frac{10}{100} \times 10 + \frac{80}{100} \times 80 + \frac{10}{100} \times 10\right] = 0.66 \qquad (3.4)$$

So in this particular table *all* the observed agreement might simply be due to chance. On the other hand, the agreement to be expected by chance in Table 3.8 is given by

$$P_c = \frac{1}{100}\left[\frac{40}{100} \times 30 + \frac{30}{100} \times 40 + \frac{30}{100} \times 30\right] = 0.33 \qquad (3.5)$$

which is considerably lower than the observed agreement.

Several authors have expressed opinions on the need to incorporate chance agreement into the assessment of inter-observer reliability. The clearest statement in favour of such a correction has been made by Fleiss (1975), who suggests an index which is the ratio of the difference in observed and chance agreement to the maximum possible excess of observed over chance agreement,

Table 3.7 Hypothetical data showing 66% agreement between two observers

		Observer 2			
		1	2	3	
	1	1	8	1	10
Observer 1	2	8	64	8	80
	3	1	8	1	10
		10	80	10	100

Table 3.8 Further set of data showing 66% agreement between two observers

		Observer 2			
		1	2	3	
	1	24	13	3	40
Observer 1	2	5	20	5	30
	3	1	7	22	30
		30	40	30	100

that is $1 - P_c$. This defines the well-known kappa statistic

$$\kappa = \frac{P_0 - P_c}{1 - P_c} \tag{3.6}$$

If there is complete agreement between the two raters so that all the off-diagonal cells of the table are empty, $\kappa = 1$. If observed agreement is greater than chance, then $\kappa > 0$. If observed agreement is equal to chance, $\kappa = 0$. Finally, in the unlikely event of the observed agreement being less than chance, $\kappa < 0$ with its minimum value depending on the marginal distribution.

For the data in Table 3.6, the kappa coefficient is calculated as

$$\kappa = \frac{0.64 - 0.27}{1 - 0.27} = 0.50 \tag{3.7}$$

But what constitutes good agreement? One, possibility is to judge using the 'benchmarks' provided by Landis and Koch (1977). These are given in Table 3.9. Any series of standards such as these are, of course, necessarily subjective. Nevertheless they may be helpful in the informal evaluation of a series of kappa values, although replacing numerical values with poorly defined English words may *not* be to everybody's taste.

But for many investigators, informal evaluation of observed kappa values will not be sufficient, and they may instead require tests of particular hypotheses (for example, that the population value of kappa is zero), or a procedure for assessing whether two population values differ. Additionally, confidence intervals for kappa may be required. All of these requirements depend on finding the variance of an observed value of kappa; this has been derived

Table 3.9 Evaluation of observed
kappa values

κ	Strength of agreement
0.00	Poor
0.00–0.20	Slight
0.21–0.40	Fair
0.41–0.60	Moderate
0.61–0.80	Substantial
0.81–1.00	Almost perfect

under a number of different assumptions by several authors including Everitt (1968) and Fleiss *et al.* (1969). The large sample variance of kappa, useful in setting confidence intervals or in comparing two independent kappa values, is estimated from the following rather horrendous expression:

$$
\mathrm{Var}(\kappa) \;=\; \frac{1}{n(1-P_c)^4}\Bigg\{ \sum_{i=1}^{c} p_{ii}[(1-P_c)-(p_{.i}+p_{i.})(1-P_0)]^2
$$
$$
+(1-P_0)^2 \sum_{i=1}^{c}\sum_{\substack{j=1\\ i\neq j}}^{c} p_{ij}(p_{.i}+p_{j.})^2
$$
$$
-(P_0 P_c - 2P_c + P_0)^2 \Bigg\} \tag{3.8}
$$

where p_{ij} represents the proportion of observations in the ij th cell of the table of counts of agreements and disagreements for the two observers, and $p_{i.}$ and $p_{.j}$ are the row and column marginal proportions. c is the number of rows and columns in the table.

To find the variance of the kappa value calculated for Table 3.6, it is helpful to find first the proportions, etc., needed in expression (3.7); these are given in Table 3.10. The required variance is found to be

$$
\mathrm{Var}(\kappa) = 0.00312 \tag{3.9}
$$

So an approximate 95% confidence interval is

$$
(0.387,\ 0.610) \tag{3.10}
$$

The concept of a chance corrected measure of agreement can be extended to situations involving more than two observers; for details see Fleiss and Cuzick (1979) and Schouten (1985). A *weighted* version of kappa is also possible, with weights reflecting differences in the seriousness of disagreements. In the investigation involving the classification of biopsy slides by pathologists, for example, a disagreement involving one pathologist rating a slide 'negative' and another rating it 'invasive carcinoma' would be very serious and given a high weight. An example of the calculation of weighted kappa and some comments about choice of weights are given in Dunn (1989).

Table 3.10 Classification of biopsy slides by two pathologists; terms needed for the calculation of the variance of κ

		Pathologist 2				
		1	2	3	4	5
Pathologist 1	1	0.186	0.017	0.017	0.000	0.000	0.220
	2	0.042	0.059	0.119	0.000	0.000	0.220
	3	0.000	0.017	0.305	0.000	0.000	0.322
	4	0.000	0.008	0.119	0.059	0.000	0.186
	5	0.000	0.000	0.025	0.000	0.025	0.050
		0.228	0.101	0.585	0.059	0.025	0.998

3.3.2 Measuring reliability of quantitative variables

A useful way in which to introduce the concept of reliability for a quantitative variable is via a simple *statistical model* for the observations. So let x represent the observed value of some variable of interest for a particular individual. If the observation was made a second time, say some days later, it would almost certainly differ to some degree from the first recording. A model for the observations is to assume that there is an underlying 'true' value, t, which the measuring instrument is seeking to record, but this differs from the observed value by some amount, e, which is the *measurement error*. Consequently the observed value is given by

$$x = t + e \tag{3.11}$$

In the population of subjects or patients under investigation, t is assumed to have a distribution with mean, μ, and variance, σ_t^2. The error terms are assumed to vary about a mean of zero with variance, σ_e^2. A consquence of this model is that the variability in the observed values is a combination of true score variance and error variance. A quantity that reflects the relative magnitude of the two *components* of variance, is the *intraclass correlation coefficient*, R, given by

$$R = \frac{\sigma_t^2}{\sigma_t^2 + \sigma_e^2} \tag{3.12}$$

which can be rewritten as

$$R = \frac{1}{1 + \sigma_e^2/\sigma_t^2} \tag{3.13}$$

As σ_e^2/σ_t^2 decreases, so that error variance forms a decreasing part of the variability in the observations, R increases, its upper limit of one being achieved when the error variance is zero. In the reverse case, when σ_e^2 forms an increasing portion of the observed variance, R decreases to a lower limit of zero, reached when *all* the variability in the measurements results from the error term in (3.10). The intraclass correlation coefficient can be directly interpreted as the proportion of variance of an observation due to between-subject variability in the true scores.

Interest in using R as a measure of reliability generally involves the situation in which each of a number of observers (or measuring instruments) records the value of some characteristic of interest on a number of subjects. In such a case, a slightly more complicated model is needed to represent the observations, a term being added to (3.10) to allow for differences between raters. The new model becomes

$$x = t + o + e \tag{3.14}$$

The quantity o represents a randomly selected rater's effect on an observation, assumed to vary about zero with variance σ_o^2. The three terms, t, o and e are assumed independent of one another, so that the variance of an observation is given by

$$\sigma^2 = \sigma_t^2 + \sigma_o^2 + \sigma_c^2 \tag{3.15}$$

The intraclass correlation coefficient correspondingly becomes

$$R = \frac{\sigma_t^2}{\sigma_t^2 + \sigma_o^2 + \sigma_e^2} \tag{3.16}$$

The estimation of R involves a two-way analysis of variance of the observers' by subjects' scores. To illustrate, the data shown in Table 3.11 (suggested by the example given in Dunn, 1989), will be used. These data are derived from computer-aided tomographic scans (CAT scans) of the heads of 25 psychiatric patients (see Turner *et al.,* 1986). The primary aim of such scans is to determine the size of the brain ventricle relative to that of the patient's skull (the ventricle–brain ratio or VBR = [ventricle size/brain size] × 100). For a given scan or 'slice' the VBR is determined from measurements of the perimeter of a patient's ventricle together with the perimeter of the inner surface of the skull. These measurements can be made in two ways, using either a hand-held planimeter on a projection of the X-ray image (PLAN), or from an automated pixel count based on the image displayed on a television screen (PIX). Table 3.11 gives the logged VBRs from single scans of 25 patients. The first three columns correspond to repeated determinations based on planimeter measurements, the last three columns to repeated determinations using the pixel count approach.

Summary statistics (means and standard deviations), for the measurements are given in Table 3.12, along with the Pearson product-moment correlation value for each pair of measurements. Scatterplots of each pair of measurements arranged in lower triangular form are shown in Figure 3.1

The means and standard deviations of the three PIX measurements are lower than those of the three PLAN recordings, and correlations between PIX 1, PIX 2 and PIX 3 are somewhat higher than those for PLAN 1, PLAN 2 and PLAN 3. Correlations betweeen the PIX and PLAN measurements are lower than those for the repeated PIX and PLAN measurements.

The general form for the analysis of variance of such 'raters × patients' data is shown in Table 3.13. The expected mean squares shown in this table give rise to the following unbiased estimators for the three components of variance in (3.14)

$$\hat{\sigma}_t^2 = \frac{\text{PMS} - \text{EMS}}{r} \tag{3.17}$$

$$\hat{\sigma}_o^2 = \frac{\text{RMS} - \text{EMS}}{n} \tag{3.18}$$

Table 3.11   CAT scan data (logged VBRs) on 25 patients

PLAN 1	PLAN 2	PLAN 3	PIX 1	PIX 2	PIX 3
2.05	2.13	2.10	1.79	1.77	1.81
1.72	1.28	1.83	1.53	1.55	1.54
1.93	1.79	1.65	1.57	1.57	1.56
2.16	1.96	2.01	1.65	1.70	1.60
2.27	1.95	1.78	2.05	2.12	2.10
2.53	2.17	2.40	2.03	1.98	2.16
1.79	1.67	1.80	1.63	1.65	1.67
1.87	1.48	1.90	1.51	1.49	1.50
1.57	1.57	1.60	1.69	1.79	1.62
1.39	1.39	1.43	1.50	1.55	1.53
1.89	1.84	1.75	1.74	1.72	1.81
2.39	2.26	2.18	1.95	1.89	1.93
1.67	1.72	1.71	1.74	1.77	1.78
1.57	1.39	1.45	1.67	1.69	1.69
2.30	2.25	2.18	1.91	1.74	1.81
2.03	1.93	2.08	2.03	1.99	2.00
1.19	1.70	1.61	0.88	0.96	1.00
1.13	0.41	0.75	1.25	1.28	1.27
1.63	1.22	1.71	1.79	1.77	1.81
1.93	2.03	1.95	1.84	1.89	1.78
1.89	1.50	1.82	1.22	1.22	1.24
1.63	2.03	1.71	1.90	1.99	1.91
1.70	1.96	2.01	2.11	2.15	2.07
2.82	2.84	2.87	2.19	2.03	2.01
0.53	0.99	1.01	1.10	1.19	1.21

Table 3.12   Means, standard deviations and correlations of PLAN and PIX recordings

Measurement	Mean	Standard deviation
PLAN 1	1.82	0.48
PLAN 2	1.74	0.48
PLAN 3	1.81	0.42
PIX 1	1.69	0.32
PIX 2	1.70	0.30
PIX 3	1.70	0.30

	Correlation matrix					
	PLAN 1	PLAN 2	PLAN 3	PIX1	PIX 2	PIX 3
PLAN 1	1.00					
PLAN 2	0.81	1.00				
PLAN 3	0.89	0.90	1.00			
PIX 1	0.74	0.70	0.69	1.00		
PIX 2	0.65	0.64	0.60	0.98	1.00	
PIX 3	0.70	0.66	0.64	0.98	0.97	1.00

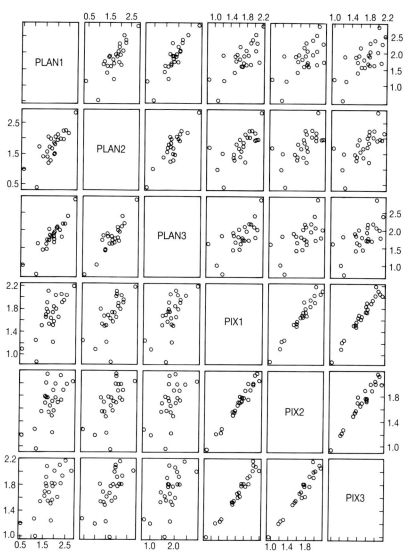

Figure 3.1 Scatterplots of PLAN and PIX measurements

$$\hat{\sigma}_e^2 = \text{EMS} \qquad (3.19)$$

The estimator of the intraclass correlation coefficient is then simply

$$\hat{R} = \frac{\hat{\sigma}_t^2}{\hat{\sigma}_t^2 + \hat{\sigma}_o^2 + \hat{\sigma}_e^2} \qquad (3.20)$$

For the data in Table 3.11 the analyses-of-variance tables for the PLAN and PIX measurements are shown in Tables 3.14 (a) and 3.14 (b). Taking first the results for the planimeter recordings, the following estimates of the variance

Table 3.13   Analysis of variance table for reliability study

Source of variation	d.f.	MS	Expected mean square
Patients	$n-1$	PMS	$\sigma_e^2 + r\sigma_t^2$
Raters	$r-1$	RMS	$\sigma_e^2 + n\sigma_o^2$
Error	$(n-1)(r-1)$	EMS	σ_e^2

r = number of raters
n = number of patients

Table 3.14   Analysis of variance tables for PLAN and PIX measures

(a) PLAN Source of variation	d.f.	MS
Patients	24	0.57848
Raters	2	0.05285
Error	48	0.03003

(b) PIX Source of variation	d.f.	MS
Patients	24	0.27825
Raters	2	0.00036
Error	48	0.00239

components are found, $\hat{\sigma}_t^2 = 0.182817, \hat{\sigma}_o^2 = 0.0009128, \hat{\sigma}_e^2 = 0.03003$, leading to an estimated intraclass correlation coefficient of 0.855.

Examining now Table 3.14 (b), the corresponding variance component estimates are $\hat{\sigma}_t^2 = 0.09195, \hat{\sigma}_o^2 < 0, \hat{\sigma}_e^2 = 0.00239$. Here, since the error mean square is *greater* than that due to raters, $\hat{\sigma}_o^2$ is negative. Usually, in the estimation of R, the value would be set to zero, leading here to $\hat{R} = 0.975$. These data suggest that the pixel method is considerably more reliable than the older planimetry-based procedure.

In the case of two raters, rating say n subjects, the intraclass correlation is equivalent to the Pearson product-moment correlation between $2n$ pairs of observations, the first n of which are the original recordings, and the second n the original observations in reverse order. Again when only two raters are involved, the value of R depends in part on the corresponding product-moment correlation, but is also dependent on the differences between the means and the standard deviations of the two sets of ratings. It can be show that R and R_{pm} (the product-moment coefficient) are related by the following formula:

$$R = \frac{[s_1^2 + s_2^2 - (s_1 - s_2)^2]R_{pm} - (\bar{x}_1 - \bar{x}_2)^2/2}{s_1^2 + s_2^2 + (\bar{x}_1 - \bar{x}_2)^2/2} \tag{3.21}$$

where $\bar{x}_1$ and $\bar{x}_2$ are the mean values of the ratings of observer 1 and observer 2 (or instrument 1 and instrument 2), and s_1 and s_2 the corresponding standard deviations.

Sample sizes required in reliability studies concerned with estimating the intraclass correlation coefficient are discussed in Donner and Eliasziw (1987), and the same authors (Eliasziw and Donner, 1987), also consider the question of the optimal choice of r and n that minimizes the overall cost of a reliability study. Their conclusion is that an increase in r for fixed n provides more information than an increase in n for fixed r.

3.4 Summary

Medical investigations often involve measurements of different types ranging from the simplest improved/not improved scale through ordinal to interval and ratio scales. Clearly all such measurements or observations need to be made as accurately as possible, and investigators need to pay careful attention to checking the reliability of their measuring instruments before undertaking any analysis of the recordings made. In this chapter only a brief account of the assessment of reliability in particular situations has been given. More detailed descriptions are to be found in Fleiss (1986) and Dunn (1989).

4

Statistical Inference

4.1 Introduction

For many clinicians the *raison d'être* of the statistician is to perform various standard calculations after the data have been collected, and deliver the verdict *significant* or *non-significant*. More enlightened members of the medical profession may accept that the statistician can also be useful in the design and planning stage of a study, but even these often regard the application of statistical significance tests as the statistician's major contribution to a piece of 'collaborative' research. The medical literature is littered with the results of *t*-tests, chi-square tests, Mann–Whitney *U*s and the like, and in addition, many of the tables in such journals are liberally 'decorated' with *, ** or even ***, to indicate varying degrees of statistical significance. (Sprent, 1970, has commented that this type of 'star' nomenclature is more suited to a hotel guide-book than a serious scientific paper.) Whether such enthusiasm for the ubiquitous significance test is entirely justified will be discussed later in this chapter, and alternatives, such as estimation and confidence intervals, will be described. Related topics such as power, sample size determination, interim analysis and meta analysis will also be considered.

As mentioned in Chapter 1, it will be assumed that readers are familiar with the most common types of significance test, for example those mentioned above, and additionally with concepts such as type I and type II errors; consequently details of those will not be of concern. The main aim of this chapter is to give an overview and a brief critique of significance tests, along with some practical advice on their use in the context of medical investigations, particularly clinical trials. (A much fuller discussion of the philosophy behind significance tests is given in the excellent text of Oakes, 1986.)

4.2 Testing hypotheses — the significance test

After learning how to calculate a mean and standard deviation, and how to construct a histogram, a clinician's next contact with statistics is very likely to involve a significance test, usually the *t*-test or chi-square test. Often this early exposure to such tests is the start of a lifelong affair, with their use becoming so routine that medical researchers rarely stop to consider whether the tests are appropriate for a particular situation or, indeed, if they are the most useful way of assessing results. Many investigators still seem to feel (despite numerous comments to the contrary — see later) that the presence of such tests is essential for their study and subsequent papers to achieve scientific respectability.

One of the problems is that medical researchers continue to use significance tests irrespective of the type of sample, type of research problem, or type of research design. Often they make important technical errors in the application of the tests (see White, 1979) but worse, many still appear to cling to a *p* value of 0.05 as if it were sacred, and continue to use the language of acceptance and rejection even when the empirical phenomena under investigation are continuous in nature. Such an approach to significance testing has been criticized frequently in the literature see for example, Rozenboom (1960) and Oakes (1986). The following quotation from Skipper *et al.* (1967) concisely summarizes such criticisms.

> The current obsession with 0.05, it would seem, has the consequence of differentiating significant research findings from those best forgotten, published studies from unpublished ones, and renewal of grants from termination. It would not be difficult to document the joy experienced by a social scientist when his *F*-ratio or *t*-value yields significance at 0.05 nor his horror when the table reads 'only' 0.10 or 0.06. One comes to internalize the difference between 0.05 and 0.06 as 'right' versus 'wrong,' 'creditable' versus 'embarrassing, 'success' versus 'failure.'

It would clearly be in their interests if clinicians could be persuaded to think in terms of 'support', 'lack of support', 'weak support', 'strong support', etc. when assessing results, since in science, adjustment of degree of belief based on the strength of evidence, rather than firm decision, is the appropriate response to the analysis of any set of observations.

Oakes (1986) presents some results which indicate that although significance tests are very familiar to most researchers and used in almost every paper presenting research findings, the general degree of understanding of the true meaning of the results of such tests is very low. Evidence that this is so was produced when Oakes put the following test to 70 academic psychologists.

> Suppose you have a treatment which you suspect may alter performance on a certain task. You compare the means of your control and experimental groups (say 20 subjects in each sample). Further suppose you use a simple independent means *t*-test and your result is $t = 2.7$ d.f. $= 18$, $p = 0.01$. Please mark each of the statements below as true or false.

Table 4.1 Frequencies and percentages of 'true' responses

Statement	f	%
1. The null hypothesis is absolutely disproved	1	1.4
2. The probability of the null hypothesis has been found	25	35.7
3. The experimental hypothesis is absolutely proved	4	5.7
4. The probability of the experimental hypothesis can be deduced	46	65.7
5. The probability that the decision taken is wrong is known	60	85.7
6. A replication has a 0.99 probability of being significant	42	60.0

(Reproduced with permission from Oakes, 1986).

(1) You have absolutely disproved the null hypothesis that there is no difference between the population means,
(2) You have found the probability of the null hypothesis being true,
(3) You have absolutely proved your experimental hypothesis,
(4) You can deduce the probability of the experimental hypothesis being true,
(5) You know, if you decided to reject the null hypothesis, the probability that you are making the wrong decision,
(6) You have a reliable experiment in the sense that if, hypothetically, the experiment were repeated a great number of times, you would obtain a significant result on 99% of occasions.

The subjects were all university lecturers, research fellows or postgraduate students. The results presented in Table 4.1 are illuminating.

Under a relative frequency view of probability all six statements are in fact *false*. Only 3 out of 70 subjects came to this conclusion. The correct interpretation of the probability associated with the observed *t*-value is:

the probability of obtaining the observed data (or data that are more extreme) if the null hypothesis were true.

Clearly the number of false statements described as true in this experiment would have been reduced if the true statement had been included with the six others. Nevertheless the exercise was extremely interesting in highlighting the misguided appreciation of significance tests held by a group of research psychologists. It seems likely that similar misconceptions might be held amongst medical researchers.

It is, of course, important to differentiate between statistical and substantive or clinical significance. The former should not be taken by investigators to be especially noteworthy regardless of any clinical importance (although it very often is!). On the other hand a marginally non-significant result (at some arbitrary level such as 0.05) should not simply be disregarded if the results suggest something that might be clinically interesting. Such over emphasis on hypothesis testing and the use of *p* values to dichotimize results into significant and non-significant is *not* recommended, and indeed has detracted from more useful procedures for interpreting the results from medical investigations such as *estimation* and *confidence intervals*, topics discussed in the next section.

4.3 Estimation and confidence intervals

Gardner and Altman (1986) make the point that the excessive use of hypothesis testing at the expense of other ways of assessing results has reached such a degree that levels of significance are often quoted alone in the main text and abstracts of papers, with no mention of actual concentrations, proportions, etc., or their differences. The implications of hypothesis testing — that there can always be a simple 'yes' or 'no' answer as the fundamental result from a medical study — is clearly false, and used in this way hypothesis testing is of limited value.

The alternative to presenting results in terms of *p* values, in relation to a statistical null hypothesis, is to estimate the magnitude of some parameter of interest along with some interval which includes the population value of the parameter with some specified probability. Such *confidence intervals* can be found relatively simply for many quantities of interest (see Gardner and Altman, 1986, for details) and although the underlying logic of interval estimates is essentially similar to that of significance tests, they do not carry with them the pseudo scientific hypothesis testing language of such tests. Instead they give a plausible range of values for the unknown parameter, with, for example, inadequate sample size being signalled by the sheer width of the interval. As Oakes (1986) rightly comments:

> [T]he significance test relates to what the population parameter is *not*: the confidence interval gives a plausible range for what the parameter *is*.

4.4 Power and sample size

One of the most frequent questions faced by the statistician acting as advisor to medical researchers is 'how many patients do I need?' Whatever type of statistical design is used for a study, this question of sample size is fundamental. Practical, ethical and statistical issues are all involved in determining the sample size needed for an investigation. Considering first the ethical issues, a study with too many subjects may be deemed unethical through the unnecessary involvement of extra people. Such studies are rare. On the other hand, studies with samples which are too small will be unlikely to detect clinically important effects. Such investigations are also usually regarded as unethical in their use of patients and other resources, although with the emergence of meta-analysis (see later) and the increasing appreciation that few studies can involve sufficient patients to resolve important clinical questions, the categorical assertion that trials with low statistical power are unethical may be outdated. Even so, studies which are too small are, unfortunately, only too common. Andersen (1990), for example, reports a study from the *New England Journal of Medicine*, in which 52 patients with severe cirrhosis and variceal haemorrhage requiring six or more units of blood were randomly assigned either to sclerotherapy or portocaval shunt. There was no difference in short term survival, with 13 patients in the sclerotherapy group discharged alive, as compared with ten patients in the shunt group. The authors commented as follows 'We failed to demonstrate any significant difference in long-term survival .... endoscopic sclerotherapy is at least as good as, and may well be better than, definitive early surgical shunting.' The absence of any significant difference made the investigators conclude that one treatment is at least as effective as the other. They failed to consider the possibility of an error of the second kind. A trial with 26 patients in each group has only a 50–50 chance of a significant outcome if the true survival rate on one treatment is 25% and on the other twice as much. Even though more patients were discharged alive after sclerotherapy than after portocaval shunt, it is possible that the operation might eventually turn out to be superior.

Further examples of the possible problems caused by inadequate sample sizes is provided by Freiman *et al.* (1978), who looked at 71 published trials with 'negative' results, defined as having *p* values greater than 0.1. By constructing confidence intervals for each study they found that nearly half the studies were compatible with a 50% therapeutic improvement, a value likely to be of clinical importance in most cases. The lack of a statistically significant result in these investigations could be the result of the small sample sizes and the consequent lack of *power* of the significance tests.

The power of a test is defined as the probability that the test will lead to rejection of the null hypothesis in favour of the alternative when the null hypothesis is indeed false. In any particular situation the power is a function of three factors:

(1) the significance level adopted,
(2) the reliability of the sample data,
(3) the size of the treatment effect.

The statistics of sample size determination are essentially based on the concept of power. The investigator needs to specify the size of the treatment difference it is important to detect and with what degree of certainty, that is with what power. Given such information the calculation of the required sample size is often relatively straightforward, although the details will depend on the type of response variable and type of test involved. In many cases tables are available which enable the required sample size to be simply read off. Examples are given in Cohen (1977) and Kraemer and Thiemann (1987). Additionally computer software is now available for determining sample size — see, for example, SOLO power analysis, BMDP Statistical Software Inc. (1992).

As an example of the calculations involved in sample size determination consider a study involving the comparison of two treatments for anorexia nervosa. Anorexic women are to be randomly assigned to one of the two treatments and the gain in weight in kilograms after three months is to be used as the outcome measure. From previous experience gained in similar trials it is known that the standard deviation of weight gain is likely to be about 4 kg. The investigator feels that a difference in weight gain in the two treatment groups of 4 kg would be of clinical importance, and wishes to have a power of 0.90 when the appropriate one-tailed test is used with significance level, $\alpha = 0.05$.

The null and alternative hypotheses here are

$$H_0 : \mu_1 = \mu_2$$
$$H_1 : \mu_1 > \mu_2$$

where μ_1 and μ_2 are the population means of weight gain for the two treatments. Assume that the population variance of weight gain is the same for both treatments, having the value $\sigma^2 = 16.0\text{kg}^2$. If the same number of subjects are to be used in each group then the appropriate test statistic is given by

$$z = \frac{\bar{x}_1 - \bar{x}_2}{\sigma} \frac{\sqrt{n}}{\sqrt{2}} \tag{4.1}$$

where $\bar{x}_1$ and $\bar{x}_2$ are the average weight gains observed in the two-treatment groups. The null hypothesis is rejected in favour of the alternative if

$$z > z_\alpha \tag{4.2}$$

where z_α is the appropriate normal deviate (here where $\alpha = 0.05, z_\alpha = 1.64$). The type II error, β, is defined to be

$$\beta = P(\text{accepting } H_0 | H_1 \text{ true}) \tag{4.3}$$
$$= P(z < z_\alpha | H_1 \text{ true})$$

If H_1 is true then z has a normal distribution with mean given by

$$\mu = \frac{\mu_1 - \mu_2}{\sigma} \frac{\sqrt{n}}{\sqrt{2}} \tag{4.4}$$

and variance equal to one. Therefore

$$\beta = P(z < z_\alpha | z \sim N(\mu, 1)) \tag{4.5}$$

So that

$$\beta = \int_{-\infty}^{z_\alpha - \mu} \frac{1}{\sqrt{2\pi}} e^{-x^2/2} dx \tag{4.6}$$

Additionally

$$\beta = \int_{-\infty}^{z_\beta} \frac{1}{\sqrt{2\pi}} e^{-x^2/2} dx \tag{4.7}$$

Consequently

$$z_\beta = z_\alpha - \mu \tag{4.8}$$

Leading to

$$\frac{\mu_1 - \mu_2}{\sigma} \frac{\sqrt{n}}{\sqrt{2}} = z_\alpha - z_\beta \tag{4.9}$$

and

$$n = \frac{2(z_\alpha - z_\beta)^2 \sigma^2}{(\mu_1 - \mu_2)^2} \tag{4.10}$$

In the example involving the trial of anorexic women, $\sigma^2 = 16.0, \mu_1 - \mu_2 = 4.0, z_\alpha = 1.64$ and $z_\beta = -1.28$, so that $n = 17$ patients are required for each treatment. (If the investigator planned to use a two-tailed test then z_α in (4.10) would need to be replaced by $z_{\alpha/2}$).

A problem with this approach is that of choosing suitable values for σ and $\mu_1 - \mu_2$. If there is little or no past data on patient variation for the chosen response variable it may be impossible to choose a realistic value for σ. Choosing a sensible and clinically relevant value for the difference, $\mu_1 - \mu_2$, may also not always be straightforward.

In many medical investigations the outcome measure of most interest will be dichotomous, for example, improved or not improved, dead or alive at end of study, etc. The main interest becomes that of assessing whether there is a difference in, say, the probability of improving in the two treatment groups. The usual test involved is the simple chi-square, and it is easy to show that the number of patients needed to detect a difference, $p_1 - p_2$, with power $1 - \beta$ when testing at the α level is

$$n = \frac{p_1(1 - p_1) + p_2(1 - p_2)}{(p_2 - p_1)^2}(z_\alpha - z_\beta)^2 \qquad (4.11)$$

As an example of the use of (4.11) consider a study in which the investigator is concerned with detecting a difference between $p_1 = 0.80$ and $p_2 = 0.50$ with a power of 95%, when testing at the 5% level. Here $z_\alpha = 1.64, z_\beta = -1.64$ and $n = 49$.

The formula in (4.11) gives the required sample size when using the chi-square test statistic *without* the continuity corrrection. Fleiss (1973) gives the corresponding formula and relevant tables for use when a continuity correction is to be applied. An alternative to the chi-square test which is often used is Fisher's exact test. Suitable tables for determining sample size in this case are provided by Cassagrande *et al.* (1978).

A very useful graphical device for calculating sample size in a variety of different situations is provided by Altman (1982, 1991). This diagram is shown in Figure 4.1. The left hand scale of the diagram involves the *standardized difference*, essentially the ratio of the difference of interest to the standard deviation of the observations. The right hand scale represents power. To determine the sample size required for a particular standardized difference, a particular power and a particular significance level (5% or 1%), a line is drawn from the appropriate point on the left hand axis to the selected power on the right and the sample size is read from the line corresponding to the chosen significance level. (The sample sizes given are for two-tailed tests). So, for example, in the anorexia trial, the standardized difference was 1.0, and the required power 0.90. Using Figure 4.1 the value of n is found to be 40, that is 20 subjects in each treatment group.

(A comprehensive review of sample size estimation in clinical trials is given in Donner, 1984.)

4.5 Interim analyses in clinical trials

In most clinical trials patients are entered one at a time and their responses to treatment observed sequentially. As data accumulates investigators may use it to check, amongst other things, protocol compliance and the incidence

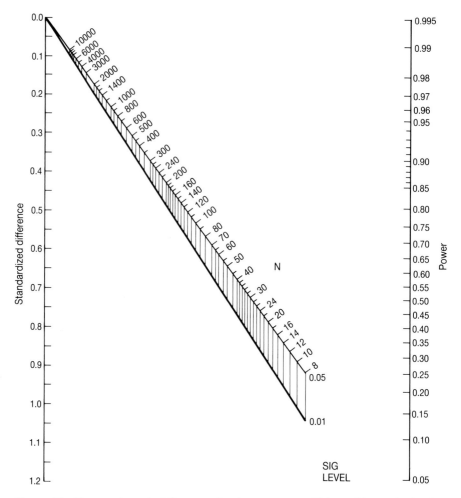

Figure 4.1   Diagram for calculating sample size or power.   (Taken with permission from Altman, 1991.)

of adverse side effects. Such checks are clearly sensible and non-contentious. Interim analyses are, however, most often used to look for treatment differences which are large and convincing enough to terminate or change the trial at a stage earlier than originally planned, the rationale being, of course, to ensure that the maximum number of patients receive the most effective treatment. Whilst it is obviously ethically desirable to terminate a clinical trial early if one therapy is clearly better than the alternative under test, interim analyses are rarely straightforward and often raise difficult statistical problems, of which the most important is that involving the use of repeated tests of significance. If on each analysis the usual test of the treatment difference for the particular situation involved is applied, then inappropriate rejection of the null hypothesis will occur more often than with a single final analysis. In other words, repeated

Table 4.2 Repeated significance tests on accumulating data

Number of repeated tests at the 5% level	Overall significance level
1	0.05
2	0.08
3	0.11
4	0.13
5	0.14
10	0.19
20	0.25
50	0.32
100	0.37
1000	0.53
∞	1.0

(Taken with permission from S. J. Pocock, *Clinical Trials* 1983, John Wiley & Sons Ltd.)

interim analyses increase the probability of a type I error. Armitage *et al.* (1969) discuss this problem and derive the actual significance levels corresponding to various numbers of interim analyses. These values are shown in Table 4.2. So, for example, if five interim analyses were performed, the chance of at least one showing a treatment difference significant at the 5% level, when the null hypothesis of no treatment difference is true, is 0.14.

Clearly the frequency of testing needs to be taken into account when carrying out interim analyses and the significance levels must be adjusted in some way. McPherson (1982) and Pocock (1978) for example, both suggest the use of a more stringent *nominal significance level* for each repeated test, in an effort to keep the overall significance level at the required value of say, 0.05 or 0.01. Table 4.3 shows the nominal significance levels required for various numbers of interim analyses. If, for example, ten interim analyses are planned during a trial (and such analyses should be *planned* rather than carried out in a capricious fashion), each test needs to be performed at approximately the 1% level to retain an overall type I error of 5%. In some cases the significance level of the test performed at each interim analysis need not necessarily be kept constant. A decision over whether to continue the trial or not may be taken when the first test is significant although other factors than simply the result of a significance test will need to be considered.

Adjusting significance levels when carrying out interim analyses is clearly necessary, but some suggested procedures can lead to inconsistencies. Falissard and Lellouch (1991), for example, consider a trial planned with four interim analyses and a final one, each analysis occurring after a constant number of patients in each group. A z test is scheduled for each group step, the overall type I error α being equal to 0.05. Pocock's method rejects H_0 if for at least an i ($i = 1, \ldots, 5$) $|z_i| \geqslant 2.41$. Now suppose the results are $|z_i| < 2.41$ for ($i = 1, \ldots, 4$) and $z_5 = 2.20$; an investigator using no interim analyses will reject H_0, while one using Pocock's procedure will accept it. Thus, the two investigators will reach different conclusions with exactly the same data.

Table 4.3   Nominal significance levels required for repeated two-sided significance testing with overall significance level $\alpha = 0.05$ or 0.01 and various values of N, the maximum number of tests

N	$\alpha = 0.05$	$\alpha = 0.01$
2	0.029	0.0056
3	0.022	0.0041
4	0.018	0.0033
5	0.016	0.0028
10	0.0106	0.0018
15	0.0086	0.0015
20	0.0075	0.0013

(Taken with permission from S. J. Pocock, *Clinical Trials* 1983, John Wiley & Sons Ltd.)

Falissard and Lellouch (1991) propose a new approach which eliminates some of these inconsistencies. This requires, for rejecting the null hypothesis, that a succession of r tests are significant at the current α level. The value of r is chosen so that the global type I error probability is also near to α.

If interim analyses are to be part of a clinical trial the investigator planning the trial needs to consider both how many such analyses there should be and how many subjects should be evaluated between successive analyses. The questions are considered in detail by Pocock (1983) and McPherson (1982). These authors also provide tables showing power and expected sample sizes for trials with various numbers of interim analyses. For large values of the treatment difference the expected sample size is considerably reduced by many interim analyses. In most trials however such large differences are unlikely, and in these circumstances Pocock (1983) suggests that there is little statistical advantage in having a large number of repeated significance tests. As a general rule Pocock recommends a maximum of five interim analyses. (Other aspects of the use of interim analyses in clinical trials are discussed in Chi *et al.*, 1986.)

4.6 Meta-analysis

Contradictory results among randomised clinical trials addressing similar questions are common and occur when the conclusions of different groups of investigators disagree, or when the results of several trials are statistically inconclusive. As a result of these contradictory reports, a lively discussion has emerged as to how these conflicts should be resolved. The term meta-analysis has been used to describe the process of evaluating and combining the results of existing clinical trials.

Gerbarg and Horiwitz (1988)

Meta-analysis, sometimes called *overviewing* or *pooling*, refers to a collection of techniques whereby the results of two or more independent studies are statistically combined to yield an overall answer to a question of interest. According to Chalmers and Lau (1993) this approach has such striking advantages over the classical (and often subjective) review article that it should largely replace the latter in the medical literature. The rationale behind meta-analysis is to provide a more powerful test of the null hypothesis than is provided by the

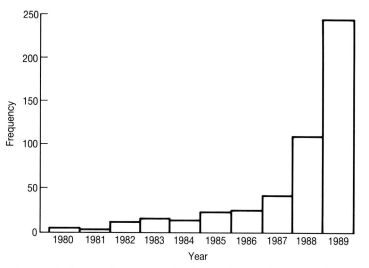

Figure 4.2 Growth of meta-analysis. (Taken with permission from Altman, 1991.)

separate studies themselves. Such an approach has become increasingly popular during the last decade or so — see Figure 4.2, taken from Altman (1991), and its use in clinical trials is reviewed in Chalmers *et al.* (1987). Meta-analysis is not without its critics but before looking at possible problems with the procedure a brief account of the statistics involved will be given, followed by a description of a recent example of the application of the method.

4.6.1 The statistics of meta-analysis

A full account of the statistical basis of meta-analysis is given in Simes (1987) and in Fleiss (1993). The main problem concerns how to combine the results from the separate studies being considered into an overall tests of a 'no treatment effect' null hypothesis. Here interest will centre on the procedure for combining measures of treatment difference (which might involve differences in means, odds ratios, etc., see Chapters 6 and 12), into a good estimator of the assumed common underlying treatment effect. As a concrete example suppose that the measure of effect size given by each of the studies included is the standardized difference between two means

$$Y = \frac{\bar{x}_1 - \bar{x}_2}{s} \tag{4.12}$$

where $\bar{x}_1$ and $\bar{x}_2$ are the means in two treatment groups and s is the square root of the pooled variance. Fleiss (1993) shows that a good combined estimator using values $Y_1, Y_2, \ldots, Y_c$ from c studies is

$$\bar{Y} = \frac{\sum_{i=1}^{c} w_i Y_i}{\sum_{i=1}^{c} w_i} \tag{4.13}$$

where

$$w_i = \frac{n_{i1} n_{i2}}{n_{i1} + n_{i2}} \tag{4.14}$$

with n_{i1} and n_{i2} being the sample sizes in each treatment group for the ith study. The standard error of $\bar{Y}$ is given by

$$SE(\bar{Y}) = \left(\sum_{i=1}^{c} w_i\right)^{-1/2} \tag{4.15}$$

The null hypothesis that the population effect size is zero may be tested with a two-tailed test by calculating the statistic

$$z = \frac{\bar{Y}}{SE(\bar{Y})} = \bar{Y}\sqrt{\sum_{i=1}^{c} w_i} \tag{4.16}$$

and rejecting the hypothesis if $|z| > z_{\alpha/2}$ where $z_{\alpha/2}$ is the $100\,(1-\alpha/2)$ percentile of the standard normal distribution. An approximate $100\,(1-\alpha)\%$ confidence interval for the population effect size, say ψ is

$$\bar{Y} - z_{\alpha/2}\bigg/\sqrt{\sum_{i=1}^{c} w_i} \leqslant \psi \leqslant \bar{Y} + z_{\alpha/2}\bigg/\sqrt{\sum_{i=1}^{c} w_i} \tag{4.17}$$

Fleiss considers the problem of assessing whether the effect sizes from the different studies are homogeneous, an obvious pre-requisite to any form of combined estimator. An appropriate test statistic is

$$Q = \sum_{i=1}^{c} w_i (Y_i - \bar{Y})^2 \tag{4.18}$$

The hypothesis of homogeneity is rejected if Q exceeds $\chi^2_{c-1,\alpha}$, the upper 100 $(1-\alpha)$ percentile of the chi-square distribution with $c-1$ degrees of freedom. If statistically significant heterogeneity is found, a single overall analysis of all studies may not be valid.

4.6.2 An example of a meta-analysis

Meta-analysis has been used to combine results from studies of beta-blockers in post myocardial infarction (Yusuf *et al.*, 1985), antibiotic prophylaxis in colon surgery (Baum *et al.*, 1981), aspirin in coronary heart disease (Breddin *et al.*, 1979), acupuncture for chronic pain (Patel *et al.*, 1989) and in many other areas. Here an example given by Fleiss (1993) will be considered. Table 4.4 gives relevant statistics from five comparative studies of the effect of psychotherapy on patients hospitalized for medical reasons. The outcome measure was, in some studies the number of readmissions to hospitals, and in other studies the number of days spent in hospital. Further details are given in Mumford *et al.* (1984).

Table 4.4 Descriptive statistics for five studies of the effect of mental health treatment on medical utilization

Study	n_1	$\bar{X}_1$	sd_1	n_2	$\bar{X}_2$	sd_2	s^*
	Psychotherapy			*Control*			
1	13	5.0	4.7	13	6.5	3.8	4.27
2	30	4.90	1.71	50	6.10	2.3	2.10
3	35	22.5	3.44	35	24.9	10.65	7.91
4	20	12.5	1.47	20	12.3	1.66	1.57
5	8	6.50	0.76	8	7.38	1.41	1.13

* s is the square root of the weighted average of sd_1^2 and sd_2^2

The weighted average of the five effect sizes is

$$\bar{Y} = \frac{20.137}{56.75} = 0.355 \qquad (4.19)$$

with an estimated standard error of

$$\text{SE}(\bar{Y}) = \frac{1}{\sqrt{56.75}} = 0.133 \qquad (4.20)$$

An approximate 95% confidence interval for ψ, the assumed common underlying effect size is

$$0.355 - 1.96 \times 0.133 \leqslant \psi \leqslant 0.355 + 1.96 \times 0.133 = (0.09, 0.62) \qquad (4.21)$$

Since the confidence interval does not include the value 0, the hypothesis that $\psi = 0$ can be rejected.

The chi-square test statistic for homogeneity given by (4.18) takes the value 3.96 with 4 degrees of freedom. There is no statistical evidence for interstudy variation in the standardized difference.

4.6.3 Problems of meta-analysis

Meta-analysis is not without its critics. Oakes (1986, 1993) is particularly sceptical, and it is clear that many problems need to be confronted if such an approach is to lead to sensible and acceptable conclusions. A fundamental question that confronts anyone who wishes to summarize a body of research is 'which studies should be included?' As Oakes (1993) comments, 'selection is a matter of inclusions and exclusions and the judgements required are problematic: should only randomised trials be included; should poor quality research be excluded; should only a single endpoint be analysed; should secondary reported results be included? And so on'. Some authors suggest a minimal entry requirement. Peto (1987), for example, suggests that only randomized trials be considered. Many meta-analysts would probably want to exclude studies which they thought were of poor quality, although Fleiss (1987), takes a different view, arguing that such studies should be included since judgements about how seriously a study is flawed are likely to be very subjective.

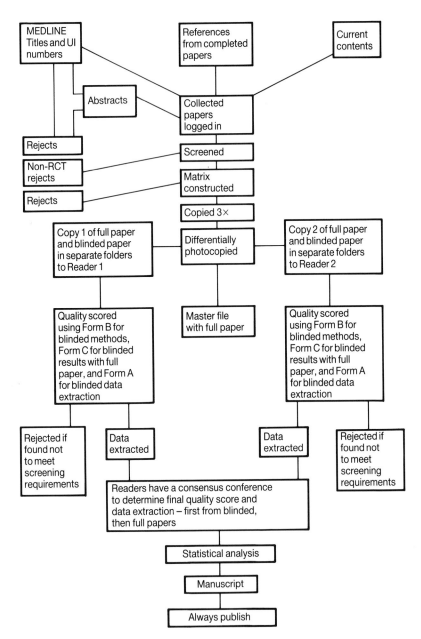

Figure 4.3 Diagram of meta-analytic process designed to ensure that all relevant published articles are included. (Taken with permission from Chalmers and Lau, 1993.)

Chalmers and Lau (1993), in an effort to overcome the opportunities provided to change the results of a meta-analysis by selecting trials whose conclusions agree with preconceived notions and rejecting those that do not, suggest the approach outlined in Figure 4.3.

A further problem with meta-analysis is that of possible publication bias. Journal articles are unlikely to be a representative sample of work addressed to any particular area of research. Published clinical trials may be biased in favour of 'significant' or of 'promising' results. Clinical trials which fail to show any treatment differences are less likely to be published owing to investigators not writing up the results or to journals declining the paper. Conclusions of the therapeutic effectiveness based on a review of only the published papers may, consequently, be seriously misleading. Rosenthal (1979) considers this problem and concludes that, in many cases, an improbable number of studies would have had to be confined to the 'file-drawer' to alter the conclusion reached from the published studies. Oakes (1993) rejects this conclusion and suggests that unpublished studies *can* cause problems for meta-analysis. Simes (1987) suggests a number of ways in which this particular criticism of the meta-analysis approach might be overcome.

Gerberg and Horiwitz (1988) argue that the criteria for judging meta-analysis should be similar to those used for judging individual randomized trials or multi-centre trials; for example, ensuring similarity at baseline for important prognostic features, equal potency and administration of the principal, comparative and ancillary therapies, equal detection of outcome events and sufficient similarity of patients to warrant combining the data from multiple centres into a single analysis. In their review of the literature on meta-analysis in medical research, Gerberg and Horiwitz find that many of the reported analyses do not meet these basic requirements. In a pooled analysis of the use of steroids as a risk factor for peptic ulcer disease, for example, one study combined 16 trials involving children with 55 studies involving adults. This illustrates the question posed in Oakes (1986, 1993), namely, to what population does the inference or estimate resulting from meta-analysis apply?

According to Chalmers and Lau (1993), 'the new scientific discipline of meta-analysis is here to stay.' Properly conducted meta-analysis are likely to be very valuable in providing practical answers to difficult and often controversial clinical questions. A good example is provided in Thompson (1993). Additionally a successful meta-analysis may remove the need for conducting further trials in a particular area. There are, however, difficulties in carrying out such analyses and a great deal of care is needed to produce unbiased and convincing results.

4.7 Summary

Statistical significance tests are commonly and widely used in medical research, although not always appropriately or wisely. In many cases, a confidence interval for a parameter is likely to be far more informative than the p value from a significance test. Small treatment effects are likely to be detectable only in studies with adequate numbers of patients, and prior estimation of sample size is an important aspect of study design. The planning of interim analyses is also an essential feature of well-designed trials that requires careful consideration of the statistical problems involved. Lastly, the combination of results from similar trials is a tempting procedure for obtaining a more powerful test of a null hypothesis. Meta-analysis is not, however, without problems and an excellent and detailed account of these is given in Begg and Berlin (1988).

5

Regression Analysis

5.1 Introduction

A frequent situation confronting the medical researcher is the detection of important prognostic variables that affect some outcome variable. The investigator might, for example, be interested in determining how response to a drug is influenced by the age and sex of a patient. The main statistical tool for such situations is some form of *regression model*. Such models are familiar from the case where a response variable and a single independent or *explanatory* variable are related by a simple *linear* regression model. In the situation where there is a quantitative response variable and several explanatory variables, the model becomes that of *multiple regression*. When the response variable is categorical, in particular binary, a commonly used approach is the *linear-logistic* model. Both multiple regression and logistic regression models are discussed in this chapter after a general introduction to regression models.

5.2 Regression models

Consider a situation where a researcher is interested in describing the number of times people visit their GP annually as a function of age. After a large set of relevant data has been analysed, suppose it is found that the average number of visits is given by the following equation

$$\text{VISITS} = 2 + \frac{1}{20} \times \text{AGE} \tag{5.1}$$

This means that, on average, a person aged 40 will visit their doctor four times a year, a person aged 80, six times and so on. The general form of equation such as (5.1) is

$$y = \beta_0 + \beta_1 x \tag{5.2}$$

where y is the response variable (in (5.1), VISITS) and x is the explanatory variable (in (5.1), AGE). The *parameters* of this model, β_0 and β_1, are the

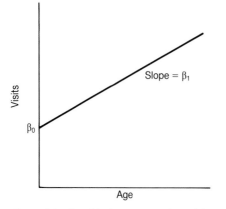

Figure 5.1   Graphical representation of the model specified by (5.2)

intercept and *slope* of the straight line represented by equation (5.2) as indicated in Figure 5.1. These parameters are often known as *regression coefficients.*

A further question of interest might be: after allowing for the effect of AGE, does a person's SEX have any bearing on the frequency of visits to a physician? On the assumption that it has, an appropriate model might be

$$\text{VISITS} = \beta_0 + \beta_1\text{AGE} + \beta_2\text{SEX} \tag{5.3}$$

or, in general

$$y = \beta_0 + \beta_1 x_1 + \beta_2 x_2 \tag{5.4}$$

This description is not quite so straightforward as before because the variable SEX cannot have the same quantitative meaning as measurements of a person's AGE. In fact it is defined to be a so-called *dummy variable* that takes a value of 0 for men and 1 for women; it is merely a way of distinguishing between males and females. The model in (5.4) now describes the two lines shown in Figure 5.2. These lines are parallel, with their common slope equal to β_1. The parameter β_0 is the intercept of the line for men on the vertical axis, and β_2 is the vertical distance between the two lines. The parameter β_2 (which could, of course, be negative), is a measure of the influence of a person's sex on the expected annual number of visits to a doctor. Here, if β_2 is positive then the model implies that women visit their doctor more often than men; if β_2 is negative then the reverse is the case. Since in this case the lines for males and females are parallel, the effect of AGE on frequency of visits is the same for both sexes, or, equivalently, the effect of a person's SEX is the same for all ages. These are merely different ways of saying that there is no *interaction* between the effects of AGE and SEX.

Suppose now that a model is required which *does* allows for the possibility of a SEX by AGE interaction on frequency of visits to a GP. Such a model needs to include a new variable, which is defined as the product of the variables AGE and SEX. The new model is therefore

$$\text{VISITS} = \beta_0 + \beta_1\text{AGE} + \beta_2\text{SEX} + \beta_3(\text{AGE} \times \text{SEX}) \tag{5.5}$$

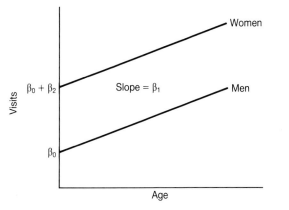

Figure 5.2 Graphical representation of the model specified by (5.4)

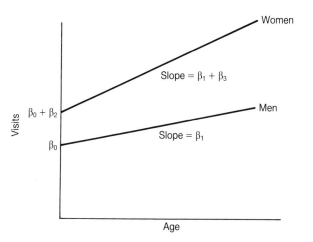

Figure 5.3 Graphical representation of the model specified by (5.7)

To understand this equation, first consider the number of visits by men. Here both the value of SEX and SEX × AGE are zero and equation (5.5) reduces to

$$\text{VISITS} = \beta_0 + \beta_1 \text{AGE} \qquad (5.6)$$

For women however, SEX = 1 and so SEX × AGE = AGE, and (5.5) becomes

$$\text{VISITS} = (\beta_0 + \beta_2) + (\beta_1 + \beta_3)\text{AGE} \qquad (5.7)$$

So the new model allows the lines for males and females to be other than parallel (see Figure 5.3). The parameter β_3 is a measure of the difference between the slopes of the two lines.

The above process is an example of *model building* and provides an approach by which a mathematical description of the relationship between the response and explanatory variables can be found. (How the parameters are estimated and how well the model fits the data are questions taken up later in this chapter.) All the models discussed above involve a *linear combination* of the parameters $\beta_0, \beta_1, \beta_2, \ldots$, and consequently are known as *linear models*. It is important to appreciate that linearity is a property of how the parameters appear in the model rather than the explanatory variables, so that the following are also regarded as linear models

$$y = \beta_0 + \beta_1 x + \beta_2 x^2 + \beta_3 x^3 \tag{5.8}$$

$$y = \beta_0 + \beta_1 x_1 x_2 + \beta_2 x_3 x_4 \tag{5.9}$$

The following are examples of *non-linear models*

$$y = e^{\beta_0 + \beta_1 x_1 + \beta_2 x_2} \tag{5.10}$$

$$y = \beta_0 + \beta_1 e^{\beta_2 x_1} + \beta_3 e^{\beta_4 x_2} \tag{5.11}$$

Some non-linear models can be converted into linear form by an appropriate transformation. In (5.10), for example, taking logs leads to

$$\ln(y) = \beta_0 + \beta_1 x_1 + \beta_2 x_2 \tag{5.12}$$

which is a linear model for $\ln(y)$. Such a transformation to linearity is not possible with (5.11).

Linear models are used far more often than those that are non-linear because they are mathematically easier to manipulate and usually easier to interpret. Fortunately they appear to provide an adequate description of many data sets. The models in equations (5.1), (5.2), etc. apply essentially to the *expected* values of the response variable. The equivalent models appropriate for observed values of the response variable need to take account of individual variation. So, for example, (5.2) would become

$$y_i = \beta_0 + \beta_1 x_i + \epsilon_i \tag{5.13}$$

where y_i is the value of the response variable for individual i and ϵ_i is a *disturbance* or *error* term reflecting the descrepancy between y_i and the expected value of the response.

5.3 Multiple regression

The data shown in Table 5.1 consist of survival times for a number of patients with multiple myeloma, along with the values of five potentially important prognostic variables. (The data are adapted from those given by Krall *et al.* 1975.) Analyses of these data would be directed primarily to discovering which of the explanatory variables has most influence on survival. In Table 5.2, body weight and various measurements of body size are given for 25 infants born in hospital. Here development of an equation useful for *predicting* body weight from the other measurements might be of most interest (see Chapter 1).

A suitable model for both situations is that of multiple regression, namely

$$y_i = \beta_0 + \beta_1 x_{i1} + \beta_2 x_{i2} + \ldots + \beta_p x_{ip} + \epsilon_i \tag{5.14}$$

where y_i and $x_{i1}, x_{i2}, \ldots, x_{ip}$ are the values of the response and explanatory

Table 5.1 Survival times for 48 patients with multiple myeloma data

Subject	y	x_1	x_2	x_3	x_4	x_5
1	1.25	2.2175	1	0	2	10
2	1.25	1.9395	1	0	1	18
3	2.00	1.5185	1	0	1	15
4	2.00	1.7482	0	13	2	12
5	2.00	1.3010	0	0	1	9
6	3.00	1.5441	1	3	2	10
7	5.00	2.2355	1	8	1	9
8	5.00	1.6812	1	1	2	9
9	6.00	1.3617	1	7	2	8
10	6.00	2.1139	0	6	2	8
11	6.00	1.1139	1	11	2	10
12	6.00	1.4150	1	10	2	8
13	7.00	1.9777	1	9	2	10
14	7.00	1.0414	0	0	2	10
15	7.00	1.1761	1	13	1	13
16	9.00	1.7243	1	4	2	12
17	11.00	1.1139	1	8	2	10
18	11.00	1.2304	1	7	1	9
19	11.00	1.3010	1	4	2	10
20	11.00	1.5682	1	5	2	12
21	11.00	1.0792	1	5	2	9
22	13.00	0.7782	0	12	2	10
23	14.00	1.3979	1	7	1	10
24	15.00	1.6021	1	16	2	11
25	16.00	1.3424	1	0	2	10
26	16.00	1.3222	1	5	2	10
27	17.00	1.2304	1	9	2	9
28	17.00	1.5911	1	1	2	10
29	18.00	1.4472	1	17	2	8
30	19.00	1.0792	1	0	2	15
31	19.00	1.2553	1	2	1	9
32	24.00	1.3010	1	12	2	9
33	25.00	1.0000	1	3	2	10
34	26.00	1.2304	1	0	1	11
35	32.00	1.3222	1	6	8	9
36	35.00	1.1139	0	16	1	10
37	37.00	1.6021	1	10	1	9
38	41.00	1.0000	1	5	1	10
39	41.00	1.4161	1	18	2	9
40	51.00	1.5682	0	10	2	13
41	52.00	1.0000	1	1	1	10
42	54.00	1.2553	1	8	1	10
43	58.00	1.2041	1	9	1	10
44	66.00	1.4472	1	4	2	9
45	67.00	1.3222	1	24	1	10
46	88.00	1.1761	1	22	1	9
47	89.00	1.3222	1	7	1	9
48	92.00	1.4314	1	12	1	11

y = survival time in days
x_1 = log blood urea nitrogen
x_2 = platelets at diagnosis: 0 = abnormal, 1 = normal
x_3 = percent lymphocytes in peripheral blood
x_4 = Bence Jones protein in urine at diagnosis: 1 = present, 2 = none
x_5 = serum calcium (mgm%) at diagnosis

Table 5.2   Birth weight, mid-arm circumference and chest circumference for 25 newly born infants

Subject	Birthweight (g)	Mid-arm circumference (cm)	Chest circumference (cm)
1	2772.8	9.2	31.8
2	2665.7	8.8	30.7
3	2794.5	9.4	31.2
4	2797.3	9.2	32.4
5	2753.5	9.6	30.4
6	2690.8	8.8	31.2
7	2590.9	8.9	31.8
8	2710.1	10.1	32.8
9	2662.7	8.6	30.8
10	2814.4	10.3	32.2
11	2679.7	9.9	30.8
12	2690.6	9.5	31.5
13	2753.5	9.1	30.7
14	2498.5	8.3	29.9
15	2673.1	9.0	31.0
16	2629.9	9.2	31.7
17	2568.2	8.9	29.8
18	2513.3	8.2	29.2
19	2706.7	8.6	31.5
20	2828.0	9.8	32.6
21	2631.9	9.3	32.0
22	2735.9	10.0	32.5
23	2721.0	10.1	32.5
24	2826.0	10.3	33.0
25	2643.9	9.7	31.7

variables for the ith individual. The error terms, $\epsilon_i, i = 1, \ldots n$, are assumed to be independently distributed with zero mean and constant variance, σ^2. (An additional assumption needed later is that the error terms are normally distributed). The x_is are assumed to be measured without error, so they are not considered to be random variables. A multiple regression model involving explanatory variables which *are* measured with error (the most common situation), is then valid only on the assumption that it is conditioned on those fixed values of the x_is actually observed. The regression coefficients $\beta_1, \beta_2, \ldots, \beta_p$ must be estimated from the sample values. The usual estimation procedure employed is *least squares*, details of which are given in Draper and Smith (1981) and Chatterjee and Price (1991). These authors also give other technical details such as how to calculate the standard errors of the estimates etc.

The regression coefficients can be interpreted as the average amount by which the response variable y changes, when the corresponding explanatory variable changes by one unit *and the other explanatory variables remain constant*. This interpretation is, however, very dependent on the implicit assumption that the explanatory variables are not strongly interrelated. If they are, it clearly becomes very difficult to imagine changing one of them whilst leaving the others fixed. If some of the explanatory variables are highly correlated it is often wise to consider removing a number of them prior to undertaking the

Table 5.3   Regression coefficients for survival time data

Variable	SD(x)	Coefficient	Standard error	Standardized coefficient
x_1	0.313	−15.257	9.157	−4.773
x_2	0.350	12.267	7.671	4.298
x_3	6.350	1.237	0.500	7.855
x_4	0.484	−22.207	6.043	−10.739
x_5	1.825	−1.879	1.593	−3.428

The constant in the regression equation is 80.914

estimation of the regression coefficients. (This difficulty is often refered to as *collinearity*.) Other possibilities for dealing with large correlations between the x_is are *ridge regression* (see Draper and Smith, 1981) and regression on principal component scores (see Chatterjee and Price, 1991).

As an illustration of the use of the multiple regression model, Table 5.3 gives the least squares estimates of the regression coefficients for the survival time data in Table 5.1, along with their standard errors. In Table 5.3, the coefficient for platelets at diagnosis, 12.267, is larger than the coefficient for percent lymphocytes, 1.237. This does not necessarily mean that platelets is a 'more important' variable than lymphocytes in determining survival time. The relative importance of variables may be compared in terms of *standardized coefficients*. The coefficient $\hat{\beta}_i$ needs to be multiplied by the standard deviation of x_i in order to obtain a coefficient in standard units. Each standardized value measures the change in the response variable resulting from a change of one standard deviation in the corresponding x variable. The standardized coefficients for the survival time data are also shown in Table 5.3 and demonstrate that lymphocytes is really a more important variable than platelets since its standardized regression coefficient is larger.

A global test for the fit of a multiple regression model is found by splitting the total variation of the response variable into a part due to regression and a residual or error term as shown in Table 5.4. The ratio

$$F = \frac{\text{MS due to regression}}{\text{MS about regression}} \tag{5.15}$$

provides a test of the null hypothesis that $\beta_1 = \beta_2 = \ldots = \beta_p = 0$, that is *none* of the explanatory variables affect the response variable. The relevant partition of the variance for the survival times data is shown in Table 5.5. Here the test statistic in (5.15) is highly significant. Clearly not all the regression coefficients are zero in this example although some of them might be. Investigating which of the prognostic variables are of most importance is taken up later.

An index of the fit of the model is provided by the proportion of the variance in the response variable accounted for by the explanatory variables, namely

$$I = (\text{TSS} - \text{RSS})/\text{TSS} = 1 - \text{RSS}/\text{TSS} \tag{5.16}$$

Another important quantity is the *multiple correlation coefficient*, R, which is simply the Pearson correlation coefficient between the response variable y and

Table 5.4   Analysis of variance table for multiple regression model

Source	d.f.	SS	MS
Due to regression	p	RGSS	RGSS/p
Residual (about regression)	$n - p - 1$	RSS	RSS/$(n - p - 1)$
Total	$n - 1$	TSS	

d.f. = degrees of freedom. *SS* = sum of squares. *MS* = mean square.

Table 5.5   Analysis of variance table for survival times regression

Source	d.f.	SS	MS	F	p
Due to regression	5	12223.64	2444.73	6.29	0.0002
About regression	42	16328.73	388.78		

its value as predicted from the values of the explanatory variables and the estimated regression coefficients, $\hat{y}$. The coefficient I is related to R as follows

$$I = R^2 \tag{5.17}$$

For the survival times data $R = 0.65$ and $I = 0.43$. The explanatory variables account for 43% of the variance of survival times.

5.3.1 Choosing important explanatory variables

The global test that all regression coefficients are zero is seldom very informative. It is likely to be significant in most applications, leading to a rejection of this very general hypothesis. The investigator is more likely to be concerned with assessing whether some subset of the explanatory variables provides an adequate description of the variation in the response variable. If a small number of the explanatory variables produces a model which fits the data only marginally worse than a larger set, then a more parsimonious description of the data results. A simpler model has several advantages, not least of which is that it eases the, at times, difficult problem of interpretation.

One possible solution to selecting a subset of explanatory variables might appear to be simply to use the standard errors of the estimated regression coefficients to test which are significantly different from zero, and then to drop the variables corresponding to those which are not. Such a procedure has limited usefulness, however, since the coefficients and their standard errors are estimated *conditional* on other variables in the model. If a variable is dropped, the remaining regression coefficients (and their standard errors), need to be re-estimated from a further analysis on the remaining variables.

More suitable procedures for identifying important subsets of explanatory variables are the so called *selection* methods, *forward selection, backward elimination* and a combination of both, known as *stepwise* regression. The criterion used for assessing whether a variable should be added to an existing model in forward selection or removed from an existing model during backward elimination is, essentially, the change in the error sum-of-squares produced by the inclusion or exclusion of a variable or subset of variables. This can be compared with the residual sum-of-squares in the complete model by a form of F test. Specifically the F-statistic is calculated as

$$F = \frac{(SS_{error,k} - SS_{error,p})/(p - k)}{SS_{error,p}/(n - p - 1)} \qquad (5.18)$$

where $SS_{error,p}$ is the residual sum-of-squares when all explanatory variables are included in the regression equation and $SS_{error,k}$, the corresponding term when only k variables are included.

The calculated F value is then compared with a preset term known as the *F to enter* (forward selection), or the *F to remove*, (backward elimination). In the former, calculated Fs greater than the *F to enter*, lead to inclusion of the variable under consideration in the current regression equation. In the latter, a calculated F less than the *F to remove*, leads to a variable currently in the regression equation being discarded. In the stepwise procedure, variables are entered as with forward selection, but after each addition of a new variable, those variables currently in the model are considered for removal by the backward elimination process. In this way it is possible that variables included at some early stage are later removed, because the presence of new variables has made their contribution to the regression model no longer significant.

In the best of all possible worlds the final model selected by each of these procedures would be identical. This does often happen, but it is in no way guaranteed. It should also be stressed that none of these automatic procedures for selecting subsets of variables are foolproof. They must be used with care, and warnings such as those given in McKay and Campbell (1982a, b), concerning the validity of the F tests used to judge whether variables should be included or eliminated, must be noted. (Other interesting methods which have been developed for selecting subsets of exploratory variables in multiple regression are discussed by Mallows, 1973 and Allen, 1971.)

The forward selection approach to choosing the most informative explanatory variables will be illustrated on the survival times data. Setting the *F to enter* to 4.0, leads to the series of steps shown in Table 5.6. Two variables from the original five, namely whether Bence Jones protein was present in the urine or not, and % lymphocytes in peripheral blood at diagnosis, are chosen as important by the forward selection procedure. The regression equation involving only these two variables is

SURVIVAL TIME $= 46.34 - 20.61\,BJP + 1.47\%$ LYMPHOCYTES (5.19)

The value of the multiple correlation coefficient is 0.58 so that 33% of the variance in survival time is accounted for by the two explanatory variables chosen by the forward selection process. Figure 5.4 illustrates graphically the fitted regression equation which consists essentially of two regression lines for survival time on % LYMPHOCYTES, one for Bence Jones protein present and one for Bence Jones protein absent.

5.3.2 Examining residuals and other diagnostics for the regression model

Multiple regression is one of the most commonly used statistical methods and it has been applied in many different disciplines. Unfortunately, as well as being one of the most used techniques it is also one of the most misused,

Table 5.6   Forward selection procedure applied to survival times data

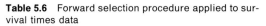

Step 0			
Variables in equation		**Variables not in equation**	
Variable	*Coefficient*	*Variable*	*F to enter*
Constant	24.43	x_4	12.02
		x_3	8.94
		x_1	3.8
		x_2	0.90
		x_5	0.98
Step 1			
Variables in equation		**Variables not in equation**	
Variables	*Coefficient*	*Variable*	*F to enter*
Constant	60.08	x_3	8.59
x_4	−22.52	x_1	3.40
		x_2	1.77
		x_5	3.67
Step 2			
Variables in equation		**Variables not in equation**	
Variable	*Coefficient*	*Variable*	*F to enter*
Constant	46.34	x_1	2.97
x_4	−20.61	x_2	2.06
x_3	1.47	x_5	1.63

Procedure stops since none of remaining variables have an *F to enter* greater than 4.0

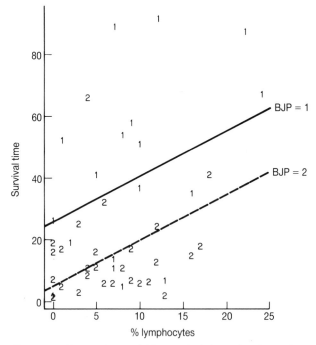

Figure 5.4   Regression model for survival times. 1 = Bence-Jones protein present; 2 = absent.

and applications frequently stop at the calculation of regression coefficients and the identification of important subsets of explanatory variables. But, in most cases, this is inadequate and the investigator needs to consider carefully the appropriateness of the models used, the assumptions of the models and problems such as the detection of outliers. This will involve the examination of a variety of *residuals* and other diagnostic indices, a number of which are considered in this section.

The basic residuals in a multiple regression analysis are simply the differences between the observed and fitted values of the dependent variable, namely

$$r_i = y_i - \hat{y}_i \tag{5.20}$$

More useful than these simple residuals are values which are standardized in a particular way (see Cook and Weisberg, 1982, for details). Various plots of these standardized residuals can be helpful in assessing particular components of the regression model. The most useful plots are:

(1) A plot of the residuals against each explanatory variable in the model. The presence of a *curvilinear* relationship, for example, suggests that a higher order term, perhaps a quadratic in the explanatory variable, should be considered for inclusion in the model.

(2) A plot of the residuals against predicted values of the response variable. If the variance of the response appears to increase with the predicted value, a transformation of the response may be in order.

(3) A normal probability plot of the residuals. After all the systematic variation has been removed from the data the residuals should look like a sample from the normal distribution. A plot of the ordered residuals against the expected order statistics from a normal distribution provides a graphical check on this assumption.

Figures 5.5 and 5.6 show plots (2) and (3) for the survival times regression specified by equation (5.18). Figure 5.5 indicates that the residuals became more variable as the predicted values increase, perhaps indicating the need for a transformation of the response variable. The normal probability plot shows some evidence of a departure from normality, suggesting once again that a transformation of the response variable might be helpful. (Since the response variable in this case is survival time, known in general to have rather a skew distribution, the assumption of normality might, *a priori*, have been considered rather unrealistic. Other perhaps more appropriate and useful models for such data are discussed in Chapter 7.)

If the regression analysis is repeated with ln(SURVIVAL TIME) as the new response variable, the previously used forward selection procedure now chooses log blood urea nitrogen, ln(BUN) and % LYMPHOCYTES as the two most informative explanatory variables, the regression equation now being estimated as

$$\text{ln(SURVIVAL TIME)} = 1.88 + 0.30\% \text{ LYMPHOCYTES} - 0.67\text{ln(BUN)} \tag{5.21}$$

The multiple correlation coefficient now takes the value 0.59. The plot of standardized residuals against predicted response and the normal probability

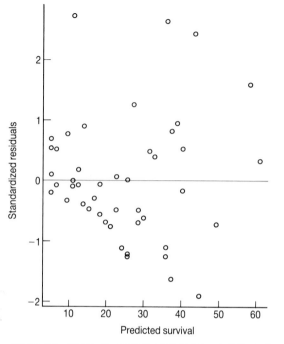

Figure 5.5 Residuals against predicted survival times for regression model fitted to myeloma data

plot for the new model are shown in Figures 5.7 and 5.8. Both plots look far more satisfactory than those for the untransformed response.

A comprehensive account of the variety of other regression diagnostics now available is given in Cook and Weisberg (1982).

5.3.3 Using the regression equation for prediction

The use of a derived multiple regression equation for prediction can be illustrated using the data in Table 5.2. The estimates of the regression coefficients for these data are given in Table 5.7. A newly born baby with mid-arm circumference, X_{ARM} and chest circumference, X_{CHEST} would have a predicted weight given by

$$\text{PREDICTED WEIGHT} = 1078.73 + 59.08X_{\text{ARM}} + 33.89X_{\text{CHEST}} \quad (5.22)$$

Clearly a prediction obtained by using this equation would be little use without a measure of its variance. The formula for the variance of a predicted value in multiple regression is given in Iles (1993). To illustrate the use of (5.22) suppose two new babies are born with arm and chest measurements (1) 10.0cm, 30.0cm and (2) 9.5cm, 29.5cm. The predicted weights of the two babies and associated confidence intervals are given in Table 5.8.

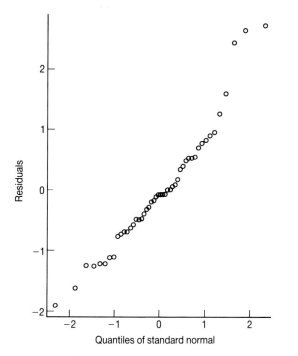

Figure 5.6 Normal probability plot of residuals for regression model fitted to myeloma data

Table 5.7 Estimates of regression coefficients for data in Table 5.2

Variable	Coefficient	SE
Mid-arm	59.08	32.66
Chest	33.89	20.05

The constant in the regression equation is 1078.73

5.4 Logistic regression

In many medical investigations the outcome variable of interest involves two states, such as, for example, responds to treatment — yes or no, or condition at end of study — improved or not improved. Table 5.9, for example, shows data from a study by Kasser and Bruce (1969) and Kronmall and Tarter (1974), involving 117 male coronary patients. Of interest here is how the variable, *history of past myocardial infarctions*, is dependent on the other variables. Data involving such a *binary* response variable are often grouped into categories before analysis. Table 5.10, for example, shows data on psychotropic drug consumption in a sample of individuals in West London, originating from a study by Murray *et al.* (1981).

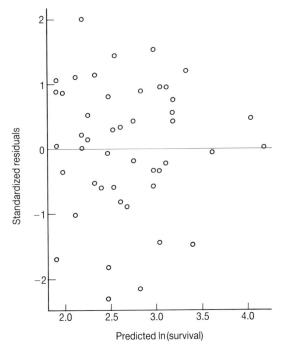

Figure 5.7   Residuals against predicted ln(survival times)

Table 5.8   Prediction of birth weight

Baby	Arm	Chest	Predicted weight	SE	95%CI
1	10.0	30.0	2686.36	6.06	2674.24–2698.48
2	9.5	29.5	2639.88	5.56	2628.75–2651.00

For such data, models for the proportion of individuals having the characteristic, or responding to treatment, etc., are of most interest, particularly to assess how this proportion, P, depends on the explanatory variables of interest. One approach would be simply to use a similar model to that considered in the previous section namely

$$P = \beta_0 + \beta_1 x_1 + \ldots + \beta_p x_p \qquad (5.23)$$

and to estimate the parameters by the usual least squares approach. Such an approach has several drawbacks however. The first is that, although the response variable in this case is constrained to be between zero and one, least squares estimation may lead to parameter estimates which give fitted values of P *outside* this range. This would clearly be unsatisfactory. A further problem is the assumption of error terms with equal variance — unlikely for this type of response (see Collett, 1991, for details). Because of such problems it is more

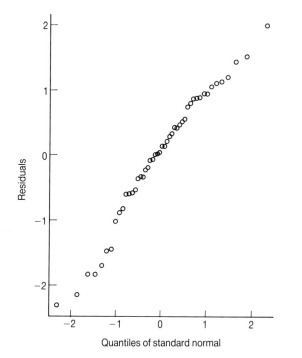

Quantiles of standard normal

Figure 5.8 Normal probability plot of residuals from regression model of ln(survival times)

useful to postulate a linear model for the response variable *after* it has been transformed in some way. The most usual (and useful) transformation for this situation is the *logistic* or *logit* defined as

$$\text{logit}(P) = \ln \frac{P}{1-P} \qquad (5.24)$$

As P varies between $(0,1)$, $\text{logit}(P)$ varies between $(-\infty, \infty)$, thus removing directly one of the problems mentioned above. The model to be fitted now becomes

$$\ln \frac{P}{1-P} = \alpha_0 + \alpha_1 x_1 + \ldots + \alpha_p x_p \qquad (5.25)$$

The parameters in this model, $\alpha_0, \alpha_1, \ldots, \alpha_p$, can no longer be estimated by least squares, but are found using an estimation procedure known as *maximum likelihood*. Details are given in Cox and Snell (1989) and Collett (1991).

Before moving on to apply the model in (5.25) to the data sets in Tables 5.9 and 5.10 it is worthwhile considering the logit transformation in a little more detail. The term $P/(1 - P)$ is the ratio of the proportion of individuals in one category of the response variable to the proportion of individuals in the other category; it is usually known as the *odds*. Consequently the logit transformation is simply log (*odds*). Also of interest in many studies is the difference in the log odds of two groups of subjects, for example, males and

Table 5.9   Infarct data

1	2	Variable 3	4	5
42	2	1	1	0
66	2	1	1	0
56	2	1	1	0
55	2	1	1	0
41	2	1	1	0
62	0	1	0	1
46	2	1	1	1
44	2	0	1	1
50	1	0	1	1
73	3	0	1	0
48	2	1	1	0
53	2	1	1	0
51	3	1	1	1
59	0	0	1	1
54	3	1	1	1
41	2	1	1	1
56	2	1	0	1
38	0	0	1	1
40	3	1	1	0
42	1	1	1	0
51	1	0	1	0
52	1	1	1	0
37	0	0	1	0
48	1	1	0	0
35	0	1	1	0
35	1	1	0	0
48	3	0	1	1
52	2	0	1	1
46	2	0	1	1
51	3	0	1	0
50	0	0	1	0
72	3	0	1	1
56	3	1	1	0
56	3	1	1	0
63	2	1	1	0
53	1	1	1	0
53	0	1	0	0
57	3	0	1	0
57	1	0	1	1
62	2	1	1	0
73	2	0	1	0
44	2	0	1	0
63	3	1	1	0
59	1	0	1	0
51	1	1	0	0
52	3	1	0	0
64	0	1	0	0
53	2	1	0	0
58	1	0	1	0
53	0	1	1	1
58	2	0	1	0
45	1	1	1	1
42	3	0	1	0
60	2	0	1	1
34	1	1	0	1
64	2	1	1	0
35	1	1	0	1
42	2	0	1	1
53	2	1	0	0
58	1	1	0	1
38	1	0	1	0
35	2	1	1	0
34	2	1	1	0

Table 5.9 Infarct data *cont.*

1	2	Variable 3	4	5
68	3	1	1	0
49	3	0	1	0
55	2	0	1	1
58	0	1	1	0
43	2	1	1	0
39	2	0	1	0
66	3	0	1	1
50	2	1	1	0
45	3	0	1	0
53	0	0	1	0
56	3	1	1	1
49	2	1	1	1
49	0	1	0	0
56	2	1	1	0
38	0	1	1	0
39	0	1	1	0
62	2	1	1	0
70	3	1	1	1
53	2	1	1	1
68	2	1	1	0
50	2	0	0	1
46	2	0	1	0
58	3	1	1	0
57	2	0	0	0
55	3	1	0	0
52	0	1	1	0
61	2	0	0	0
45	2	0	0	0
51	2	1	1	0
55	3	1	1	1
51	1	0	1	0
46	1	1	1	0
69	1	0	1	0
51	3	1	1	1
49	1	0	1	1
58	3	1	1	0
38	3	1	1	0
50	1	1	0	0
38	1	1	1	0
58	1	1	0	0
69	0	0	1	0
66	0	0	1	0
49	2	0	1	0
62	0	1	1	0
44	0	0	1	1
58	3	1	1	0
45	2	1	1	0
58	3	1	1	0
54	2	1	1	0
55	2	1	1	1
68	2	1	1	0
68	2	1	1	0
47	1	1	1	1
55	0	0	1	0

Variable 1 = age in years

2 = function—functional class: none (0), minimal (1), moderate (2), more than moderate (3)

3 = infarct—history of past myocardial infarctions: none (0), present (1)

4 = angina—history of agina pectoris: none (0), present (1)

5 = high bp—history of high blood pressure: none (0), present (1)

Table 5.10   Patterns of psychotropic drug consumption in a sample of individuals from West London (from Murray *et al.*, 1981)

SEX	AGE GROUP	PSYCH. CASE	Number on drugs	Total
Male	1	No	9	531
Male	2	No	16	500
Male	3	No	38	644
Male	4	No	26	275
Male	5	No	9	90
Male	1	Yes	12	171
Male	2	Yes	16	125
Male	3	Yes	31	121
Male	4	Yes	16	56
Male	5	Yes	10	26
Female	1	No	12	588
Female	2	No	42	596
Female	3	No	96	765
Female	4	No	52	327
Female	5	No	30	179
Female	1	Yes	33	210
Female	2	Yes	47	189
Female	3	Yes	71	242
Female	4	Yes	45	98
Female	5	Yes	21	60

females. This difference

$$\ln \frac{P_1}{1 - P_1} - \ln \frac{P_2}{1 - P_2} = \ln \frac{P_1(1 - P_2)}{P_2(1 - P_1)} \tag{5.26}$$

is the log of the *odds ratio*, a term dealt with more fully in Chapter 12. Lastly, if $l = \text{logit}(P)$ then

$$P = \frac{e^l}{1 + e^l} \tag{5.27}$$

The last equation is useful for interpreting the estimated regression coefficients from the logistic model as will be seen later.

As the first example of the use of the logistic regression model, it will be applied to the data in Table 5.9. The results are given in Table 5.11. The variable, FUNCTION, with four categories has been recoded in terms of three dummy variables in the following way

Value of FUNCTION	Dummy variables D1	D2	D3
0	0	0	0
1	1	0	0
2	0	1	0
3	0	0	1

Table 5.11 Logistic regression results for data in Table 5.9

Variable	Coefficient	SE	Coefficient/SE
AGE	−0.017	0.02	−0.80
ANGINA	−1.51	0.69	−2.20
FUNCTION 1	0.14	0.65	0.22
2	0.57	0.57	1.01
3	0.84	0.64	1.31
HIGH BP	−0.38	0.43	−0.90
CONSTANT	2.43	1.37	1.78

If this recoding was not used and FUNCTION was entered into the model simply as a single variable with values 0, 1, 2 and 3, it would imply the assumption that changes from, for example, 0 to 1 and 2 to 3, have an equal effect on the response variable. This is unlikely to be the case and the use of the dummy variables allows a more appropriate assessment of the effect of FUNCTION.

Comparing the estimated coefficients to their standard errors suggests that only ANGINA is important in the model. As with multiple regression however, this simple approach to assessing explanatory variables can be misleading, and some form of stepping procedure is once again used to choose important subsets of explanatory variables. With logistic regression the usual criterion for selecting variables for inclusion in the model, is the change in the *likelihood function*, a function of the observations used in the estimation process — see Collett (1991) for details. If the procedure is applied here, the only explanatory variable selected is ANGINA, which gives an improvement in the likelihood from a model containing none of the explanatory variables, equivalent to a chi-square of 4.78 with 1d.f., which is significant beyond the 5% value. The estimated model is

$$\text{logit}(P) = 1.674 - 1.302\text{ANGINA} \qquad (5.28)$$

where P is the population proportion of people having a past history of myocardial infarct. P can also be regarded as the probability of a person having had an infarct in the past. So for those patients with *no* previous history of angina, that is ANGINA = 0, the estimated model becomes

$$\text{logit}(P_0) = 1.674 \qquad (5.29)$$

where P_0 is the probability of an infarct for patients with no angina.

For patients *with* a previous history of angina, that is ANGINA = 1, the estimated model is

$$\text{logit}(P_1) = 1.674 - 1.302 \qquad (5.30)$$

where P_1 is the probability of an infarct for patients with angina

Subtracting (5.30) from (5.29) gives

$$\text{logit}(P_0) - \text{logit}(P_1) = 1.302 \qquad (5.31)$$

Table 5.12   Logistic regression results for data in Table 5.10

(1) *Details of stepwise procedure*

Step number	Variable entered	Chi-square	d.f.	Improvement chi-square	d.f.
0		467.18	19		
1	CASE	243.05	18	224.13	1
2	AGE	59.77	14	183.28	4
3	SEX	14.32	13	45.46	1

(2) *Estimated regression coefficients etc.*

Variable	Coefficient	SE	Coeff/SE	Exp(coeff)	LCI	UCI
SEX	0.63	0.09	6.57	1.87	1.55	2.26
AGE 1	0.77	0.16	4.77	2.16	1.57	2.96
2	1.31	0.15	8.88	3.71	2.78	4.96
3	1.74	0.16	10.70	5.68	4.13	7.80
4	1.70	0.19	8.95	5.48	3.77	7.95
CASE	1.41	0.09	15.6	4.11	3.44	4.91

LCI = lower limit of 95% confidence interval
UCI = upper limit of 95% confidence interval

leading to

$$\frac{P_0(1 - P_1)}{P_1(1 - P_0)} = e^{1.302} = 3.68 \qquad (5.32)$$

The estimated odds ratio in (5.32) indicates that the odds of patients without a previous history of angina suffering an infarct are over three times that of patients with a previous history of agina. The confidence interval for the odds ratio can be found via the corresponding interval for the estimated regression coefficient of ANGINA. The standard error of the estimated coefficient is 0.66 and so an approximate 95% interval for the regression coefficient is $1.302 \pm 2 \times 0.66$, giving $(-0.02, 2.62)$. The 95% confidence interval for the odds ratio in (5.32) is found by simply exponentiating these two limits to give (0.991, 13.6). This includes the value one, a value corresponding to no difference between the two categories of the ANGINA variable with respect to the response variable. There seems little real evidence for a substantial effect of ANGINA. Since only 19 of the 117 patients have no previous history of angina, this is, perhaps, not too surprising.

Moving on to the data in Table 5.10, the results of fitting a logistic regression model using a stepwise procedure to choose important prognostic variables, gives the results shown in Table 5.12. All three explanatory variables appear to contribute to the model. (Note that AGE GROUP has been coded in terms of four dummy variables in a similar way as was FUNCTION in the previous example.) The fitted model is

$$\text{logit}(P) = -4.00 + 0.63\text{SEX} + 1.41\text{CASE} + 0.77D_1 + 1.31D_2 + 1.74D_3 + 1.70D_4 \qquad (5.33)$$

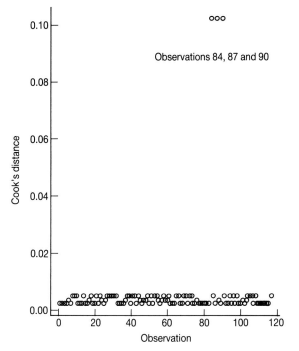

Figure 5.9 Index plot of Cook's distances for logistic regression model fitted to infarct data

where D_1, D_2, D_3 and D_4 are dummy variables coding AGE GROUP. For the youngest age (AGE GROUP = 1) all the dummy variables are zero. For SEX the estimated odds ratio *conditional* on the other variables remaining constant is 1.87 with a 95% confidence interval of (1.55,2.26). The odds of taking psychotropic drugs in women is between about one and a half and two and a quarter that of the odds in men. Similarly the odds amongst those people considered a probable psychiatric case is between about 3.5 and 5.0 times that of people not regarded as likely psychiatric cases.

There are several types of residuals and model diagnostics which can be used in logistic regression. A comprehensive account of these is given in Collett (1991). Here the use of a particular diagnostic known as *Cook's distance* will be illustrated. Essentially this index assesses how the ith observation affects the set of parameter estimates, by comparing the vector of parameter estimates for the full data set, with the vector of estimates obtained when the observation is excluded. The formula for the index is given in Collett (1991). A useful way of displaying the Cook's distances for the complete set of observations is via an *index plot,* which is simply a plot of observation number against the appropriate value of Cook's distance for the observation. Such a plot for the myocardial infarction data is shown in Figure 5.9. For the bulk of the observations the value of the diagnostic index is very small, but observations 84, 87 and 90 have considerable higher values. Returning to the original data shows that these patients are the only ones having no previous history of angina and *no history of previous myocardial infarctions.* For these

Table 5.13   Details of stepwise procedure for
ordered logistic regression example

Variable entered	d.f.	Improvement chi-square	p
ln(VOUT2)	1	111.10	0.00
ln(VOUT1)	1	7.58	0.01
SURG	1	7.61	0.01
OLD	1	7.76	0.01

data, removal of these three observations leads to problems when fitting the logistic regression model since no information is now available on one of the combinations of ANGINA with the response variable.

Green (1984), Koch and Edwards (1988), Upton (1978) and McCullagh (1980) discuss a variety of ways in which the logistic regression model can be extended to include categorical response variables with more than two categories. Two approaches which seem useful in practice are to assume first that the response variable is purely nominal, say with J categories, and fit the model

$$P[y = j] = \frac{e^{u_j}}{1 + \sum_{i=1}^{J-1} e^{u_j}}, j = 1, 2, \ldots, J - 1$$

$$P[y = J] = 1 - \sum_{j=1}^{J-1} P[y = j] \qquad (5.34)$$

where u_j is a linear function of the explanatory variables.

If the values of the response variable are considered ordinal, then a suitable model is

$$P[y > j] = \frac{e^{u_j}}{1 + e^{u_j}} \qquad (5.35)$$

for $j = 1, 2, \ldots, J - 1$ and $P[y > J] = 0$. Here the proportion of occurrences higher then the jth level is estimated.

The model in (5.35) will be illustrated with an example taken from the *BMDP Statistical Software Manual, Volume 2*, concerned with the location (LOC) of deep vein thrombosis (DVT) according to four ordered categories:

0 = No DVT,
1 = DVT in the vicinity of the ankle,
2 = DVT in the calf
3 = DVT in the thigh.

The seven explanatory variables of interest were:
1. Old Thrombosis (OLD)
2. Age (AGE)
3. Swelling (SWELL)
4. History of Previous Surgery (SURG)
5. Heparin Treatment (HEPARIN)
6. Venous Outflow 1 Second After Removing Leg Cuff (VOUT 1)
7. Venous Outflow 2 Seconds After Removing Leg Cuff (VOUT 2)
(The last two variables were transformed by taking logarithms before analysis).

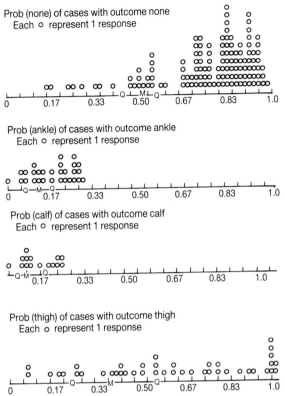

Figure 5.10 Histograms of estimated probabilities from ordered logistic regression model

A stepwise procedure identified OLD, SURG, log (VOUT 1) and log (VOUT 2) as the important explanatory variables with the estimated (by maximum likelihood) model being

$$P[\text{LOC} > \text{None}] = \frac{\exp(2.492 + D)}{1 + \exp(2.492 + D)}$$

$$P[\text{LOC} > \text{ANKLE}] = \frac{\exp(1.360 + D)}{1 + \exp(1.360 + D)}$$

$$P[\text{LOC} > \text{CALF}] = \frac{\exp(0.5669 + D)}{1 + \exp(0.5669 + D)} \qquad (5.36)$$

where

$$D = 2.182\text{OLD} + 0.9469\text{SURG} + 4.710\ln(\text{VOUT1}) - 10.64\ln(\text{VOUT2}) \quad (5.37)$$

Table 5.13 shows the improvement measure and the overall goodness-of-fit as each explanatory variable is added to the model. Figure 5.10 shows the histograms of predicted probabilities for each category of the response variable. These show that it would be possible to allocate patients to the categories NONE and THIGH, with some confidence for many individuals. Allocation to the two intermediate categories would, however, be less certain.

5.5 Summary

The identification of important prognostic variables is an essential area of medical research. When the response variable is quantitative, ideally normally distributed, the multiple regression model may be used. When the response variable is binary, the logistic model is more appropriate. Various automatic procedures are available for selecting the most useful subset of explanatory variables. Of major importance in any regression analysis is the examination of residuals and other diagnostic indices for checking model assumptions.

6

Crossover Designs, Repeated Measures Analysis of Variance and Analysis of Covariance

6.1 Introduction

One of the most commonly used classes of statistical technique in medical research is the *analysis of variance*. All members of the class are concerned with testing hypotheses about the equality of a set of means on some response variable of interest. An investigator may, for example, wish to assess whether diet affects heart rate, and randomly allocates a number of subjects to each of several different diets. In the case of just *two* diets the appropriate test to compare the heart rates of the two groups would be an independent samples *t*-test. For an investigation involving more than two diets, the *one-way analysis of variance* would be appropriate to test the equality of means in this *randomized group design*; such a procedure represents a direct extension of the *t*-test to situations involving more than two groups. *Two-way* and higher order designs which allow the simultaneous effects of two or more factors on the response variable to be assessed (in the example above, sex of subject may be a second factor of some importance). In addition, such designs make it possible to investigate the possible *interaction* between factors, that is, effects over and above the simple additive combination of the individual factors. Special types of designs such as *latin squares, balanced incomplete blocks*, etc., are also useful in particular circumstances and are described in detail in, for example, Cochran and Cox (1966).

In this chapter, a number of aspects of the analysis of variance of particular importance in medical investigations are considered. The first of these involves *repeated measures designs*, where subjects are observed on a number of different occasions. Such studies are often also referred to as *longitudinal*. An apparently simple special case of a repeated measures design, in which each subject receives two treatments, one on each of two different visits, one group of subjects having the treatments in one order, and another group having them in the reverse order, will be considered first.

The second topic to be discussed in this chapter is the *analysis of covariance*. This method is appropriate when it is required to eliminate the effect(s) of some concomitant variable (or variables), the *covariates*, on the response variable before proceeding to test hypotheses about sets of means of the variable.

6.2 Crossover designs

The simple randomized groups study, in which subjects are allocated at random to each of a number of treatments under investigation, is perhaps, the most widely used analysis of variance design in medical research. With such a design each subject receives only *one* of the possible treatments. Although this type of design has several advantages, particularly that of simplicity, it may not be attractive in the early stages of a clinical investigation where the number of subjects available is likely to be limited. Consequently it becomes of interest to consider possible alternative procedures which might be used with a smaller number of subjects to obtain a relatively precise estimate of treatment effect. One such possibility is the *crossover design*, in which each subject receives a sequence of treatments, with the treatment effect being estimated from *within-subject* comparisons. This will often allow more sensitive testing of the treatment difference than can be obtained from comparisons *between subjects*, where variation is likely to be more substantial.

6.2.1 The 2 × 2 crossover design

The simplest type of crossover design involves two treatments given to each subject on different occasions. One group of subjects receives the two treatments in one order, and a second group receives them in the reverse order. The two sequence groups are generally formed by random allocation. Clearly such an approach is only applicable to chronic conditions for which short-term relief of symptoms is the goal, rather than a cure. Typical examples of areas in which a crossover design has been used are investigations of anti-inflammatory drugs in arthritis, hypotensive agents in hypertension and treatments for asthma.

There are two main advantages to the 2 × 2 crossover design (2 groups, 2 occasions); the first is possible economy in number of subjects, since each provides two observations on response to treatment. The second is that comparisons can be made within subjects and are, consequently, affected by within-subject rather than between-subject error variation. This is likely to allow a more precise comparison of the two treatments. Such apparent advantages may, however, turn out to offer inadequate compensations for the possible disadvantages associated with this type of design that are discussed later.

The type of analysis appropriate for a 2 × 2 crossover study depends on the type of response variable involved. The two types most commonly encountered, quantitative and binary, will be considered here, beginning with the former.

Table 6.1 shows data collected during an investigation of two drugs for the treatment of patients with bronchial asthma. The response variable in the study was forced expiratory volume in one second (FEV). The data are described in detail in Patel (1983) and Kenward and Jones (1987). Patients were divided randomly into two groups, with those in the first group receiving

Table 6.1 2×2 crossover trial of single oral doses of two active drugs (A and B) in patients with bronchial asthma: forced expiratory volume in one second

Subject	Sequence Group 1 (AB)	
	Period 1	Period 2
1	1.28	1.33
2	1.60	2.21
3	2.46	2.43
4	1.41	1.81
5	1.40	0.85
6	1.12	1.20
7	0.90	0.90
8	2.41	2.79

Subject	Sequence Group 2 (BA)	
	Period 1	Period 2
9	2.68	2.10
10	2.60	2.32
11	1.48	1.30
12	2.08	2.34
13	2.72	2.48
14	1.94	1.11
15	3.35	3.23
16	1.16	1.25

the treatments in the order AB and those in the second group receiving B followed by A.

The main interest in this study will be in the assessment and estimation of the difference between the two treatments. Before the appropriate testing and estimation procedures can be derived, however, it is necessary to consider what other effects might be present and what would be a suitable model on which to base the analysis. For the 2×2 crossover design, there are two other possible effects that need consideration, in addition to that for the treatment difference. The first corresponds to the possibility that the response variable changes over time *irrespective* of the treatment given. Such a change is usually referred to as a *period* effect. A further possibility is that any difference between the two treatments varies in the two periods of testing, that is, there is a *treatment* × *period* interaction. Several possible causes of such an effect will be discussed in detail later, but perhaps the most important is the possibility that at least part of the effect of the treatment given during the first observation period *remains* during the second period, and that this *residual* or *carryover* effect is different for the two treatments.

The various possible effects may be accommodated in the following model for the data:

$$y_{ijk} = \mu + \pi_k + \phi_u + \lambda_v + \omega_{ij} + \epsilon_{ijk} \tag{6.1}$$

where y_{ijk} represents the value of the response variable for the jth subject in the ith group, in the kth period, with $j = 1, \ldots, n_i, i = 1, 2$ and $k = 1, 2$; n_i

Table 6.2 Analysis of variance table for data in Table 6.1

Source	SS	d.f.	MS	F	p
Groups	2.02	1	2.02	2.24	0.1567
Error	12.63	14	0.90		
Occasion	0.03	1	0.03	0.45	0.5135
Group × Occasion	0.25	1	0.25	4.04	0.0640
Error	0.86	14	0.06		

represents the number of subjects in group i. The terms on the right-hand side of (6.1) represent the possible influences on the response variable.

μ = overall mean,

π_k = effect of the kth period, $k = 1, 2$,

ϕ_u = effect of the uth drug, $u = A, B$,

λ_v = residual effect of the vth drug in the first period on the response in the second period, $v = A, B$, ($\lambda_v = 0$ for all first-period measurements).

ω_{ij} = effect of the jth subject in the ith group

ϵ_{ijk} = within-subject residual or error terms for the kth period.

Complete technical details of the model may be found in Brown (1980). The model in (6.1) is usually described as a *mixed model*, since the first four terms are assumed to represent *fixed* effects and the last two *random* effects. (See Winer, 1971, for more details of mixed models).

A straightforward analysis of variance table resulting from using the model in (6.1) for the asthma data in Table 6.1, is given in Table 6.2. In this table, the F ratio corresponding to the 'between-groups' term, is a test of the treatment × period interaction. Since this is not significant it can be assumed that there is no differential carryover effect of the two treatments so that λ_A and λ_B in (6.1) are equal. The F test for 'between occasions' is also non-significant so that there is no evidence of a difference in response on the two visits. Lastly the F test for the 'group × occasion' interaction term, which for the 2 × 2 crossover design represents a test of the treatment difference, does not quite reach significance at the 5% level.

The model will now be examined in more detail with a view to estimating effects of interest, particularly the treatment effect. To begin, it will be assumed that it is known *a priori* that no differential carryover effects are present, so that the terms λ_A and λ_B in (6.1) can be taken as equal.

Estimating the treatment effect: $\phi_B - \phi_A$

For each subject calculate the difference between their response values in period 1 and period 2, that is

$$D_{ij} = y_{ij2} - y_{ij1} \tag{6.2}$$

By using (6.1) and assuming that $\lambda_A = \lambda_B$, it is relatively easy to see that an estimator of the treatment effect, $\delta = \phi_B - \phi_A$, is given by

$$\hat{\delta} = \frac{1}{2}(\bar{D}_{AB} - \bar{D}_{BA}) \tag{6.3}$$

where $\bar{D}_{AB}$ and $\bar{D}_{BA}$ are the means of the differences in the two sequence groups.

The variance of $\hat{\delta}$ can be shown to be

$$V(\hat{\delta}) = \frac{1}{2}\sigma_\epsilon^2 \left[\frac{1}{n_1} + \frac{1}{n_2} \right] \tag{6.4}$$

where σ_ϵ^2 is the population variance of the random error terms in (6.1). An estimator of this variance is given by

$$\hat{\sigma}_\epsilon^2 = \frac{1}{2} \left[\frac{(n_1 - 1)s_1^2 + (n_2 - 1)s_2^2}{n_1 + n_2 - 2} \right] \tag{6.5}$$

where s_1^2 is the sample variance of the difference scores in sequence group 1, and s_2^2 is the corresponding variance for sequence group 2.

From (6.3) and (6.4) confidence intervals can be constructed for δ, and if a significance test for zero treatment effect is required, the statistic

$$t = \frac{\hat{\delta}}{\sqrt{V(\hat{\delta})}} \tag{6.6}$$

can be referred to Student's t distribution with $n_1 + n_2 - 2$ degrees of freedom.

Estimating the period effect: $\pi_2 - \pi_1$

An estimator of the period effect $\gamma = \pi_2 - \pi_1$, can also be constructed from the difference scores in each group. The estimator is

$$\hat{\gamma} = \frac{1}{2}(\bar{D}_{AB} + \bar{D}_{BA}) \tag{6.7}$$

$\hat{\gamma}$ has the same variance as $\hat{\delta}$. Consequently it is again straightforward to construct appropriate confidence intervals and test for zero period effect.

Estimating treatment and period effects for the bronchial asthma example in Table 6.1

Table 6.3 shows the difference scores for each patient in the asthma study, derived from the observations in Table 6.1. (The 'sum' scores also given in Table 6.3 will be used later). From these differences, the various terms needed to estimate the treatment and the period effect can be calculated.

$$\begin{aligned}
\bar{D}_{AB} &= 0.1175 & \bar{D}_{BA} &= -0.2350 \\
s_1^2 &= 0.1255 & s_2^2 &= 0.1203 \\
n_1 &= 8 & n_2 &= 8
\end{aligned}$$

so that

$$\hat{\sigma}_\epsilon^2 = \frac{1}{2} \left[\frac{7 \times 0.1255 + 7 \times 0.1203}{14} \right] = 0.0614$$

(Note that this is equal to the second error mean square in Table 6.2).

So that finally

$$V(\hat{\delta}) = V(\hat{\gamma}) = \frac{1}{2} \times 0.0614 \times \left[\frac{1}{8} + \frac{1}{8} \right] = 0.0767$$

Table 6.3   Difference and sum scores for the estimation of treatment, period and interaction effects for the bronchial asthma data

Subject	Sequence Group 1 (AB) Difference	Sum
1	0.05	2.61
2	0.61	3.81
3	−0.03	4.89
4	0.40	3.22
5	−0.55	2.25
6	0.08	2.32
7	0.00	1.80
8	0.38	5.20

Subject	Sequence Group 2 (BA) Difference	Sum
9	−0.58	4.78
10	−0.28	4.92
11	−0.18	2.78
12	0.26	4.42
13	−0.24	5.20
14	−0.83	3.05
15	−0.12	6.58
16	0.09	2.41

This leads to the following confidence intervals and tests for treatment and period effects

95% confidence intervals

Treatment effect	(−0.0117, 0.3641)
Period effect	(−0.2467, 0.1292)

t-tests for zero effects

Treatment	$t = 2.01, p = 0.064$
Period	$t = -0.67, p = 0.513$

(Note that the t values are simply the square roots of the appropriate F values in Table 6.2, and that the p values are identical. The two analyses are essentially equivalent.)

The results clearly show that the period effect is not significant. The difference between the two treatments just fails to reach significance at the 5% level, but gives some indication that treatment B produces a higher level of the response variable on average.

The treatment and period effect estimates and tests given above assume no differential carryover effect. If such an effect *is* present, the estimates of both treatment and period effects will be biased. So consideration now needs to be given to estimating and testing the carryover effect.

Estimating and testing the carryover effect: $\lambda_B - \lambda_A$

First the sum of the period 1 and period 2 measurements for each subject are calculated.

$$d_{ij} = y_{ij1} + y_{ij2} \tag{6.8}$$

These 'sums' are given in Table 6.3.

Again using (6.1) it is not difficult to see that an estimator of the differential carryover effect, $\alpha = \lambda_B - \lambda_A$ is given by

$$\hat{\alpha} = (\bar{d}_{BA} - \bar{d}_{AB}) \tag{6.9}$$

The variance of $\hat{\alpha}$ can be shown to be

$$V(\hat{\alpha}) = (4\sigma^2 + 2\sigma_\epsilon^2) \left[\frac{1}{n_1} + \frac{1}{n_2} \right] \tag{6.10}$$

where σ^2 is the population variance of the subject parameters in (6.1). It can be shown that the term $4\sigma^2 + 2\sigma_\epsilon^2$ in (6.10) may be estimated from

$$\frac{(n_1 - 1)s_1^2 + (n_2 - 1)s_2^2}{n_1 + n_2 - 2} \tag{6.11}$$

where now s_1^2 and s_2^2 are the sample variances of the sum scores in each sequence group.

From (6.9) and (6.10) both a confidence interval and a test for zero carryover effect can be constructed. For the asthma data the calculations involved result in the following:

$$\bar{d}_{AB} = 3.263 \quad \bar{d}_{BA} = 4.267$$
$$s_1^2 = 1.597 \quad s_2^2 = 2.011$$

So that

$$\hat{\alpha} = (4.267 - 3.263) = 1.004$$
$$V(\hat{\alpha}) = \frac{7 \times 1.597 + 7 \times 2.011}{14} \times \left[\frac{1}{8} + \frac{1}{8} \right] = 0.451$$

This leads to a 95% confidence interval for the carryover effect of (-0.439, 2.439), and the relevant t statistic takes the value 1.50 with $p = 0.157$. (Note that the latter corresponds to the 'between-groups' test in Table 6.2.)

A useful graphical aid for detecting carryover effects, which can be used to supplement the formal test outlined above, is to plot the values of (d_{ij}, D_{ij}) for each subject, distinguishing on the plot between the members of the two sequence groups. If the shift between the groups in a horizontal direction is small, then a differential carryover effect is unlikely, and the shift between the groups in a vertical direction is a measure of the treatment effect. Such a plot for the data in Table 6.1 is shown in Figure 6.1.

In the asthma study the carryover effect was found to be non-significant. Suppose however, there had been evidence of a non-zero carryover effect. Then the previously described estimators for treatment and period effects would be biased and so could not be used. In such a case, Hills and Armitage (1979) advise that the treatment effect now be estimated from the *first period* observations only, simply as the difference in the means of the two groups.

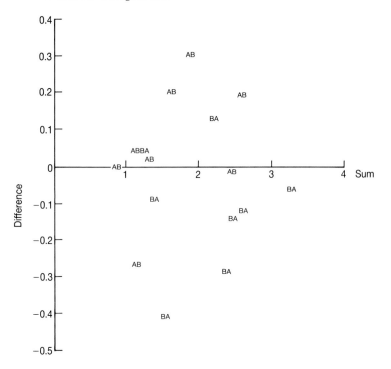

Figure 6.1 Plot of sum and difference scores for brochial asthma data

The study is thus effectively reduced to a randomized groups design. The strategy for analysis recommended by Hills and Armitage can be summarized as follows.

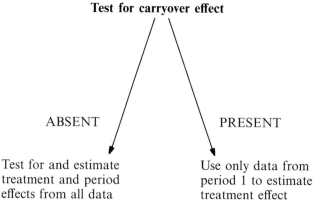

This approach appears at first sight to be reasonable. Unfortunately however, a major problem arises because the test for carryover effect, based as it is on variation *between* subjects, has low power. Consequently there is a very real chance of failing to detect a non-zero carryover effect large enough to cause substantial bias in the estimate of the treatment effect. A solution might seem to be to undertake a crossover study with sufficient power to detect even small carryover effects, with the intention of estimating the treatment effect on the basis of the first period observations only, if the test for carryover is significant. Brown (1980) demonstrates that such a procedure is unlikely to be particularly helpful, however, since to achieve a reasonable power of detecting even moderate carryover effects will require a large sample size. So to ensure a test for treatment with relatively small bias and the same power as the randomized group design, a crossover study may need up to *ten* times as many subjects. As Hills and Armitage comment

> The inescapable conclusion seems to be that a single crossover trial cannot provide the evidence for its own validity.

Clearly then it becomes of some importance to consider whether carryover effects can be dismissed on *a priori* grounds, thus making the savings in number of subjects offered by the crossover trial a practical reality. To answer this question requires a more detailed consideration of the various ways in which carryover or other interaction effects could arise. Two possibilities are as follows.

(1) A residual effect of the first treatment which remains into the second period and which is different for the two treatments. This possibility might be minimized by allowing an adequate *washout* period, this being the gap in time between the two treatment periods, during which it is hoped that the subject's clinical condition reverts, approximately at least, to its initial state. It may be possible, when the two treatments are different drugs for example, to show that the washout period has been completely effective from the *pharmacological* viewpoint, with the drug used in period 1 having been completely eliminated by the time period 2 starts. Unfortunately, however, physiological or psychological effects may persist, so that such residual effects can rarely be dismissed on *a priori* grounds.

(2) If the treatment effect varies according to the general level of the response, an interaction effect may be produced. Subjects with a greater response, for example, may show a greater treatment difference than those with a smaller response. Combined with a period effect in which period 2 scores are, on average, higher than those in period 1, this would lead to a larger treatment difference in period 2 than in period 1, leading to a period × treatment interaction.

Figure 6.2 (a) illustrates the no interaction situation, 6.2 (b) the first possibility described above, and 6.2 (c) the second possibility. It would, of course, be very difficult in most practical situations to distinguish between the possible mechanisms leading to an interaction, although Hills and Armitage (1979) offer a few potentially helpful tips.

The conclusion generally drawn from the points made above, is that the use of crossover designs is inadmissible unless the investigator is confident *a priori* that carryover effects are absent. Willan and Pater (1986) however, argue that

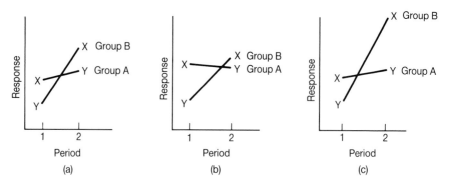

Figure 6.2   Three hypothetical outcomes in a two-period crossover design: (a) no interaction, (b) and (c) interaction

the size of carryover effect required to make the randomized group designs preferable, is substantial and, in most cases, unlikely to exist. (The use of crossover designs when *baseline* measurements are available is less dependent on *a priori* knowledge about the magnitude of carryover effects. Such studies are discussed in Section 6.2.3.)

6.2.2 Non-parametric tests for the 2 × 2 crossover design

The estimation and testing procedures detailed in the previous sections are based on the assumption that the response variable is normally distributed. In many studies involving a crossover design the number of subjects will not be large and so the assumption is difficult to check. As a result, investigators may often feel more comfortable using distribution-free tests and estimates. In such cases the Mann–Whitney test can be applied using once again the sum and difference scores of each subject as the basic data. The procedure will be illustrated on the asthma data in Table 6.1.

Testing for carryover effect

Sequence group AB: rank sum of 'sum' scores = 54.5,
    Sequence group BA: rank sum of 'sum' scores = 81.5,
    Mann–Whitney test statistic = 18.5, $p = 0.16$.

Testing for the treatment effect

Sequence group AB: rank sum of 'difference' scores = 50.0,
    Sequence group BA: rank sum of 'difference' scores = 86.0,
    Mann–Whitney test statistic = 14.0, $p = 0.06$.
    The conclusions from these tests are the same as those from the analyses reported in Section 6.2.1.
    An excellent and detailed example of the use of a non-parametric approach to the analysis of a 2 × 2 crossover design is given in Clayton and Hills (1987).

6.2.3 Crossover designs with baseline measurements

Often during a crossover trial, in addition to a washout period between the administration of the two treatments, a *run-in* period is included which

Table 6.4 2×2 crossover trial of single oral doses of two active drugs (A and B) in patients with bronchial asthma: forced expiratory volume in one second for run-in, treatment and wash-out periods

		Sequence Group (AB)		
Subject	*Run-in*	*Period 1*	*Wash-out*	*Period 2*
1	1.09	1.28	1.24	1.33
2	1.38	1.60	1.90	2.21
3	2.27	2.46	2.19	2.43
4	1.34	1.41	1.47	1.81
5	1.31	1.40	0.85	0.85
6	0.96	1.12	1.12	1.20
7	0.66	0.90	0.78	0.90
8	1.69	2.41	1.90	2.79

		Sequence Group (BA)		
Subject	*Run-in*	*Period 1*	*Wash-out*	*Period 2*
9	2.41	2.68	2.13	2.10
10	3.05	2.60	2.18	2.32
11	1.20	1.48	1.41	1.30
12	1.70	2.08	2.21	2.34
13	1.89	2.72	2.05	2.48
14	0.89	1.94	0.72	1.11
15	2.41	3.35	2.83	3.23
16	0.96	1.16	1.01	1.25

precedes the first treatment. During the run-in period both sequence groups are treated similarly being given no treatment, the standard treatment or a placebo. On the practical side such a period can serve to acclimatize the subjects to the experimental procedures. Equally importantly it can provide baseline measurements which may allow a more powerful test for interaction effects and also for the treatment effect than if this was to be based on first-period observations only.

In addition to a run-in period, a further possibility is that *second* baseline readings are taken during the washout period. Such was the situation in the trial involving the bronchial asthma patients and the complete set of data with four measurements per patient is shown in Table 6.4. The question now arises as to how the baseline measurements might be incorporated into the analysis. A number of possibilities might be considered.

Using only the run-in period baseline measurements

Let z_{ij1} represent the baseline measurement taken during the run-in period for the jth subject in the ith group. A more sensitive test for a carryover effect can now be constructed using scores given by

$$d'_{ij} = (y_{ij1} - z_{ij1}) + (y_{ij2} - z_{ij1}) \tag{6.12}$$

Incorporating the initial measurements in this way removes the between-subject variation from the comparison based simply on the period 1 + period 2 scores. If according to the test based on the values in (6.12), the carryover effect is deemed negligible, then the treatment and period effects can again be tested and estimated as described previously *without* using the baseline measurements at all, since in the absence of an interaction the previously defined estimators are optimal.

If, on the other hand, the conclusion is that a non-zero carryover effect *is* present, then the estimate and test of the treatment effect must again be confined to the first period observations only. Now however, the baseline measurements might be used to obtain more precise tests by either simply subtracting them from the first period observation and analysing the *change* scores, or alternatively using them as a *covariate* in an *analysis of covariance* (see Section 6.4). The latter may increase precision even further.

To illustrate a number of these possible approaches the data in Table 6.4 will be used, with, for the moment, the wash-out period measurement being ignored.

Test for carryover effect incorporating run-in period baseline

(1) Sequence group AB: $\bar{d}'_{AB} = 0.587, s_1^2 = 0.397$.
(2) Sequence group BA: $\bar{d}'_{BA} = 0.640, s_2^2 = 0.896$.
Leading to

$$t = 0.131, p = 0.89$$

and the conclusion that there is no carryover effect. Note that the variances of the scores defined by (6.12) are much lower than those of the simple 'sum' scores given previously.

Since the differential carryover effect is not significantly different from zero, the treatment effect would, in practice, be estimated and tested as described in Section 6.2.1, with the baseline measurements not being used. However, to illustrate the procedure adopted in the case of a significant carryover effect, the analysis of the change scores for the asthma data will be performed.

Testing for a treatment effect using first-period observations and baseline measurements

For the change scores, period one −baseline, the following can be calculated.

(1) Sequence group AB: mean 0.235, variance 0.042,
(2) Sequence group BA: mean 0.437, variance = 0.240
Giving

$$t = 1.08, p = 0.30$$

On the basis of the first period observations alone there is no evidence of a treatment effect.

Baseline measurements available for both run-in and washout periods

A comprehensive account of crossover trials with baseline measurements is given in Kenward and Jones (1987). The essential features of the model they propose are parameters, ω, θ and λ, representing respectively, the direct treatment effect, and first and second order carryover effects. The parameter θ represents any difference between the groups on the second baseline means, and λ any treatment × period interaction, whether due to carryover differences or not. Kenward and Jones show that estimators of the parameters all take the form

$$\hat{c}_1 - \hat{c}_2 \qquad (6.13)$$

where $\hat{c}_i$ is a contrast among the four means of group i, $i = 1, 2$, so that

$$\hat{c}_i = w_1 \bar{z}_{i.1} + w_2 \bar{y}_{i.1} + w_3 \bar{z}_{i.2} + w_4 \bar{y}_{i.2} \qquad (6.14)$$

where $\sum_{i=1}^{4} w_i = 0$. Any of the estimators can be defined specifically by giving the appropriate values of (w_1, w_2, w_3, w_4).

Kenward and Jones demonstrate that the parameters have different estimators depending on the assumptions that are made about the others. The estimator of the treatment effect ω, for example, when θ and λ cannot be assumed to be zero, is defined by the weights

$$(1, -1, 0, 0)$$

So the estimator of the treatment effect in this case uses only the first-period and first baseline measurements.

The estimator of θ in the presence of non-zero values of ω and λ is defined by the weights

$$\frac{1}{2}(1, 0, -1, 0)$$

Here the estimator involves differences between the two baseline measurements.

Kenward and Jones suggest that the testing and estimation procedure should begin with θ and λ, followed by the appropriate test for ω. They illustrate the procedure on the asthma data of Table 6.4.

6.2.4 Crossover designs with binary responses

Many medical investigations, including 2×2 crossover studies, involve response variables which can take only two possible 'values', for example, improved or not improved, pain relief or no pain relief, dead or alive, etc. (See also Chapter 5). Such binary variables usually have the two possible states labelled 0 and 1 for convenience. For a 2×2 crossover design the possible outcomes for a binary response can be summarized as shown in Table 6.5. An example of such a data set is shown in Table 6.6. These data arise from an investigation of two drugs in the treatment of depression, where the side effect, nausea, was of interest.

Crossover designs with binary response variables have been discussed by a number of authors including Gart (1969), Hills and Armitage (1979), Fidler (1984), and Farewell (1985). In this section a number of simple tests for assessing treatment, period and carryover effects are described. Each of these has as its basis Fisher's exact test which is described in detail in Everitt (1992). As with the discussion of the analyses appropriate for a quantitative variable, it is first assumed that there is no treatment $\times$ period interaction.

Test for treatment effect

The procedure here involves applying Fisher's exact test to the following table of frequencies

	(0, 1)	(1, 0)
Group (AB)	n_{12}	n_{13}
Group (BA)	n_{22}	n_{23}

(The theory behind the test is discussed in detail in Gart, 1969.)

Table 6.5 General form of data from a 2 × 2 crossover design with a binary response variable

Sequence group	Response (0,0)	(0,1)	(1,0)	(1,1)
AB	n_{11}	n_{12}	n_{13}	n_{14}
BA	n_{21}	n_{22}	n_{23}	n_{24}

The responses are denoted (r_1, r_2) where r_1 is the value observed in the first period and r_2 is the value in the second period.

Table 6.6 Data from a 2 × 2 crossover trial of two drugs for the treatment of depression: presence of absence or nausea recorded

Sequence group	Response (0,0)	(0,1)	(1,0)	(1,1)
AB	40	1	7	2
BA	35	6	2	7

0 = no nausea, 1 = nausea

For the data in Table 6.6 the corresponding table of frequencies is

$$
\begin{array}{ccc}
 & (0,1) & (1,0) \\
\text{Group (AB)} & 1 & 7 \\
\text{Group (BA)} & 6 & 2
\end{array}
$$

Fisher's test gives $p = 0.04$ (two-tailed) so there is some evidence of a different rate of nausea for the two drugs, with that for drug A being higher than for drug B.

Test for period effect

Now the appropriate test procedure is to apply Fisher's exact test to the following table

$$
\begin{array}{ccc}
 & \text{Nausea with A} & \text{Nausea with B} \\
\text{Group (AB)} & n_{13} & n_{12} \\
\text{Group (BA)} & n_{22} & n_{23}
\end{array}
$$

For the data in Table 6.6 the relevant table of frequencies is

$$
\begin{array}{ccc}
 & \text{Nausea with A} & \text{Nausea with B} \\
\text{Group (AB)} & 7 & 1 \\
\text{Group (BA)} & 6 & 2
\end{array}
$$

Fisher's exact test gives $p = 1.0$. Clearly no period effect exists.

Both the tests described above are strictly valid only in the absence of a treatment × period interaction. Various tests of the latter are available for binary responses. One, suggested by Hills and Armitage (1979), involves the application of Fisher's exact test to the following frequency table

	$(0,0)$	$(1,1)$
Group (AB)	n_{11}	n_{14}
Group (BA)	n_{21}	n_{24}

For the data in Table 6.6 the appropriate set of frequencies is

	$(0,0)$	$(1,1)$
Group AB	40	2
Group BA	35	7

Fisher's exact test gives $p = 0.15$, indicating that for these data there is no treatment × period interaction.

6.2.5 More complex crossover designs

The two-period, two-treatment crossover design is the one most commonly used, and the one most discussed in the literature. There are, however, a number of more complex crossover designs which have been suggested. The design with sequence groups AB, BA, AA and BB, can, for example, be used to estimate treatment effects when it is uncertain whether or not there are non-zero carryover effects. Such a design was used by Hunter *et al.* (1970) in a trial of amantadine in the treatment of Parkinson's disease.

Three-period crossover designs with two treatments are discussed by Hafner *et al.* (1988). Such designs can overcome many of the problems associated with the analysis of the two-period crossover trial. An appropriate three-period design, for example, allows for the use of *all* the data to estimate and test the direct treatment effect, even when carryover effects are present.

Reviews of crossover designs both for the two-treatment and more than two treatment situations are given by Kershner and Federer (1981), Laska *et al.* (1983), Bishop and Jones (1984) and Jones and Kenward (1989). McKnight and van den Eeden (1993), consider the problem of drop-outs (see later), in crossover trials with a binary response.

6.3 Repeated measure designs

A frequently encountered situation in clinical trials is one involving *repeated* observations of a response measure on every subject at several pre-defined times since randomization. Such post-randomization repeated measurements over time are often accompanied by one or more pre-randomization (baseline) measurements on each subject. As an example of such a data set, Table 6.7 shows observations on the Hamilton Depression Scale made during a double-blind trial of hormone replacement therapy (HRT). Women taking part in the trial were rated on this scale on two occasions prior to randomization, and then monthly for four consecutive months after treatment commenced. (Note that there are some observations missing for four women in the trial, a problem that will be addressed later.)

Table 6.7 Hamilton depression scores obtained during double-blind trial of hormone replacement therapy (HRT)

Subject	Group	BL1	BL2	V1	V2	V3	V4
1	1	11	12	11	12	15	18
2	1	5	6	7	8	7	9
3	1	11	8	8	9	10	13
4	1	10	8	10	8	12	12
5	1	2	3	5	3	M	M
6	1	7	7	10	8	9	11
7	1	5	5	7	5	6	7
8	1	7	7	7	8	9	11
9	1	10	11	13	11	14	17
10	1	3	2	2	4	3	5
11	1	7	7	8	9	10	10
12	1	7	7	9	8	11	11
13	1	3	4	5	6	6	M
14	1	5	5	5	5	7	10
15	1	7	6	8	6	9	8
16	1	4	4	5	5	M	M
17	1	9	8	10	8	11	14
18	1	2	5	5	5	7	9
19	1	6	3	4	6	4	7
20	1	5	5	5	6	7	6
21	2	1	2	4	3	0	6
22	2	8	6	7	7	10	7
23	2	4	4	2	5	6	5
24	2	8	9	8	10	9	12
25	2	2	2	3	3	3	M
26	2	4	5	5	6	4	6
27	2	3	1	2	2	2	3
28	2	9	10	10	13	9	12
29	2	8	11	12	14	11	15
30	2	6	4	1	3	8	4
31	2	2	2	3	5	1	0
32	2	1	4	1	5	1	4
33	2	8	11	13	13	10	14
34	2	4	3	5	3	6	6
35	2	5	4	6	7	8	6
36	2	2	1	1	1	1	2
37	2	7	7	8	10	8	8
38	2	5	5	7	6	6	7
39	2	4	4	3	4	2	5
40	2	5	7	7	8	6	8

Group 1 = placebo, Group 2 = active treatment
M = missing value.

There exist a number of different methods for analysing such data, ranging from the repeated use of significance tests (usually the two-sample *t*-test), at every time point, to *multivariate* analysis of variance. In the HRT study, for example, Table 6.8 shows the results of a series of *t*-tests of the between-group difference at each of the post-treatment measurement occasions. (The missing observations are simply ignored in this analysis.) According to Ekström *et al.* (1990), such an analysis was used in 32% of research studies employing

Table 6.8 *t*-tests for monthly visit depression scores in the HRT study

Visit		Placebo	Active
1	Mean	7.20	5.40
	SD	2.74	3.59
	n	20	20
	$t = 1.78, p = 0.08$		
2	Mean	7.00	6.40
	SD	2.29	3.84
	n	20	20
	$t = 0.60, p = 0.55$		
3	Mean	8.72	5.55
	SD	3.20	3.55
	n	18	20
	$t = 2.88, p = 0.01$		
4	Mean	10.47	6.84
	SD	3.59	3.97
	n	17	19
	$t = 2.86, p = 0.01$		

a repeated measures design and reported in one of four major psychiatric journals. Finney (1990) suggests that such an approach may be quite useful if the occasions are few and the intervals between them large. When, *p* values are reported without any adjustment, however, the problem of the inflation of the type 1 error rate arises (see Chapter 2), and separate analysis may be misleading. In addition such analyses give no overall answer to whether or not the treatments differ and no single measure of the treatment effect.

One alternative to a series of *t*-tests is to use an appropriate analysis of variance model for the data.

6.3.1 Analysis of variance for repeated measure designs

A suitable model for the post-treatment observations is

$$y_{ijk} = \mu + \alpha_i + \pi_k + \gamma_{ik} + \omega_{ij} + \epsilon_{ijk} \tag{6.15}$$

where y_{ijk} represents the value of the response variable for the jth subject in the ith group on the kth visit. The terms on the right hand side of (6.15) represent the various possible influences on the response variable.

μ = overall mean,
α_i = effect of the ith group $(i = 1, 2)$,
π_k = effect of the kth visit $(k = 1, 2, 3, 4)$
γ_{ik} = group $\times$ visit interaction effect,
ω_{ij} = effect of the ith subject in the jth group,
ϵ_{ijk} = residual or error term.

Full details of the model are given in Winer (1971). The terms α_i, π_k and γ_{ik} are assumed to represent *fixed* effects and ω_{ij} and ϵ_{ijk}, *random effects*, so that (6.15) is a further example of a mixed-model met earlier in the discussion of crossover trials (see equation (6.1)).

One approach to the analysis of such data would be to partition the total

Table 6.9   Analysis of variance table for post-treatment visits in HRT study

Source	SS	d.f.	MS	F	p
Between groups	211.98	1	211.98	5.12	0.03
Error	1406.58	34	41.37		
Visits	88.40	3	29.47	15.68	< 0.001
Group × Visits	42.28	3	14.09	7.50	< 0.001
Error	191.66	102	1.88		

variation in the observations into several components representing specific sources of variation as with the simple one-way and two-way designs. For the HRT data the resulting analysis of variance table is shown in Table 6.9. The F-tests indicate that the group, visits and group × visits effects are all highly significant. Interpretation of these results will be taken up later. (Only women with values for all four visits are considered in this analysis.)

It is important to consider the assumptions behind the F-tests shown in Table 6.9. These are:

(a) normality,
(b) homogeneity,
(c) compound symmetry.

The first two of these should be familiar to readers as they are the same as are made in simple analysis of variance designs. Assumption (c) is, however, unlikely to be so familiar. Essentially, compound symmetry requires that the correlations between each pair of repeated measures are equal. So in the HRT study, correlations between the observations made on each four of visits must be the same. Combined with the homogeneity requirement, compound symmetry implies that the *covariance matrix* (see Chapter 10), of the measurements has the form

$$\mathbf{V} = \begin{pmatrix} \sigma^2 & \cdots & & & \\ \rho\sigma^2 & \sigma^2 & \cdots & & \\ \rho\sigma^2 & \rho\sigma^2 & \cdots & & \\ \vdots & \vdots & \vdots & & \\ \rho\sigma^2 & \rho\sigma^2 & \cdots & \sigma^2 \end{pmatrix} \tag{6.16}$$

where ρ is the correlation between each pair of repeated measures and σ^2 is the variance of each repeated measure. The correlation and variance are assumed to be the same in each treatment group.

If the compound symmetry assumption is not valid, then neither are the F-tests in Table 6.9. The assumption might be checked by using the test suggested by Box (1950). It seems unlikely, however, that the compound symmetry will be satisfied routinely in situations involving repeated measures over time, simply because observations made at time points close to one another are likely to have higher correlations than measurements that are widely separated in time.

One approach that can be used when the compound symmetry assumption is in doubt, is to use the F-tests in Table 6.9, but with their degrees of freedom adjusted to account for the unequal correlations. Two correction factors have

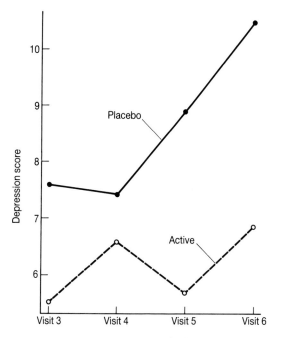

Figure 6.3 Post treatment means for HRT data

been proposed, one by Greenhouse and Geisser (1959) and one by Huynh and Feldt (1976). Both are functions of the population correlations and variances and have to be estimated from the corresponding sample statistics. (In most cases which of the two possible correction factors is used will make little difference.) The adjusted F-tests are obtained by simply multiplying the degrees of freedom by the correction factor. (This applies only to the within-subject tests since the validity of the between-group test does not depend on the compound symmetry assumption.)

For the HRT study data the correction factors are:

(1) Greenhouse and Geisser, 0.9005,
(2) Huynh–Feldt, 1.0000.

For these data the correction factors, being either at the upper limit of one, or very close to this value, lead to adjusted tests that give results which are almost identical to those in Table 6.9. Here the correlations between each pair of post-treatment visits are very similar to one another.

A plot of the post-treatment means for each group (see Figure 6.3), shows that the level of depression in each group tends to increase with time, but more rapidly in the placebo group, so that the difference between the group means varies from visit to visit. This is the reason for the significant 'groups × visits' interaction found in the original analysis of variance of the data.

Table 6.10 Analysis of mean depression scores on four post-treatment visits in HRT study

Source	SS	d.f.	MS	F	p
Groups	52.99	1	52.99	5.12	0.03
Error	351.64	34	10.34		

Estimated post-treatment difference = 2.43
Estimated variance of post-treatment difference = 1.15
Approximate 95% confidence interval = (0.284, 4.577).

An alternative approach to adjusting the degrees of freedom in the F-tests when the assumption of compound symmetry is thought not to be valid, is to use multivariate analysis of variance techniques. This method, which is described in detail in Hand and Taylor (1987), does not need the compound symmetry assumption and automatically allows for the usually heterogeneous correlations among the repeated measures. The approach does, however, have a number of disadvantages, see for example Lavori (1990), and is not widely used in medical examples of repeated measure designs.

6.3.2 The use of summary statistics in the analysis of repeated measure designs

A method often used to analyse repeated measures designs occurring in medical investigations is by the use of summary values. Such an approach is advocated by several authors including Matthews *et al.* (1989), and Frison and Pocock (1992). Essentially the procedure is to decide in advance on an *appropriate* summary of each individual's response to the treatment, and then to use simple two-group comparison techniques such as the two-sample t-test to assess treatment differences on the summary measures.

The choice of summary measures is wide, for example, the post-treatment mean, the end value, shape, maximum value, area under the curve and time to reach a peak have all been used in particular studies. In many clinical trials however, Frison and Pocock argue that the prime objective is to assess the *average* response to treatment over time, often, but not necessarily, anticipating that treatment response is likely to occur quickly and to remain reasonably steady over time. For the HRT data the analysis of the mean depression scores over the four post-treatment visits (after removing patients with missing values), leads to the results shown in Table 6.10. The between-group difference is highly significant, reflecting the difference over the four post-treatment visits seen in Figure 6.3.

The analysis can be extended to use the two pre-treatment measures by calculating for each patient the difference between the mean of the post-treatment observations and the mean of the baseline treatments. The analysis of such *change* scores is generally more sensitive than the analysis of post treatment means only (see Section 6.4). The analysis of the change scores from the HRT study is shown in Table 6.11. The estimated treatment difference is now smaller than for the post-treatment only analysis. The estimated variance of the difference is also substantially smaller than the variance of the

Table 6.11 Analysis of change scores for HRT study

Source	SS	d.f.	MS	F	p
Group	5.75	1	5.75	5.73	0.02
Error	34.08	34	1.00		

Estimated difference in change from pre-treatment = 0.800
Estimated variance of difference = 0.112
Approximate 95% confidence interval = (0.132, 1.468)

post-treatment mean difference however, and so the treatment effect remains significant at the 5% level. (A further way of using the pre-treatment measures is described in Section 6.4.)

A further type of summary value which can be useful for repeated measure designs is an estimate of the *linear trend* for each patient, or, in some cases, estimates of more complex changes over time such as *quadratic* and *cubic* trends. The relevant summaries for each patient can be calculated from what are known as *orthogonal polynomial* contrasts. In the HRT study, for example, the differences between the four post-treatment observations can be expressed in terms of a linear, quadratic and cubic trend, calculated from the original observations by applying the following series of coefficients.

	Visit			
	1	2	3	4
Linear	-3	-1	1	3
Quadratic	1	-1	-1	1
Cubic	-1	3	-3	1

If a linear trend is calculated for each subject with complete data in the HRT study and a t-test applied, the result is $t = 3.41$, $p = 0.0017$. There is a clear difference in the linear trend over the four post-treatment visits for the two groups.

6.3.3 The problem of drop-outs in repeated measures designs

One of the most difficult problems facing the researcher analysing a longitudinal clinical trial is that of patients who either drop out of the study all together, or fail to appear for one or other of the scheduled visits. In the HRT data set, for example, there are four patients with missing values. In all analyses of these data sets reported previously in this chapter, these patients have been left out.

Heyting *et al.* (1992) list the common causes of patients prematurely ceasing to participate. They are:

(1) recovery,
(2) lack of improvement,
(3) unwanted signs or symptoms that may be related to the investigational treatment,

(4)   unpleasant study procedures,
(5)   concurrent health problems,
(6)   external reasons that seem to be unrelated to the trial procedures or to the progress of the patient.

These causes may operate singly or in combination. The initiative to end participation may be taken by the patient, by the physician or jointly. It is easy to appreciate that such a variety of possible causes for drop-outs is likely to complicate the statistical analysis of such data.

Heyting *et al.* (1992) give some illustrations of how simply removing drop-outs from the analysis can produce serious bias in the assessment of treatment effect. Suppose, for example, that treatment A is modestly effective in a proportion of the patients, regardless of the initial severity of their illness, while treatment B causes the less severely ill patients to recover and leaves the severely ill patients essentially unaffected. If the recovered patients tended to drop out before the final assessment time, a simple minded comparison of an outcome measure of severity of illness for those patients completing the study, will unduly favour treatment A. The bias would be accentuated if treatment A caused some of the treatment resistant patients to drop out due to an unfavourable balance between side effects and improvement in the severity of their illness.

Different causes of patients dropping out may well result in biases in opposite directions. This would be the case if the severely ill patients receiving treatment B tended to drop out because of a combination of lack of improvement and the unpleasantness of the study procedures. In such cases, the direction of overall bias may be quite unclear.

If the number of patients who drop out is relatively small compared with the number of patients in the trial, then any biases introduced by leaving them out of the analysis are likely to be small. In many trials, however, other procedures for handling drop outs need to be considered. A number of possibilities are described in Gornbein *et al.* (1992). One which is widely used, particularly in the pharmaceutical industry, is the *last observation carried forward* method of analysis. It consists of substituting for each missing value the patient's last available assessment of the same type. Although popular, the usefulness of the method is, according to Heyting *et al.* (1992), 'very limited', since it makes very unlikely assumptions about the data.

Another more satisfactory method of dealing with missing data in repeated measure designs is via the general framework for imputing missing values suggested by Little and Rubin (1987). A maximum likelihood procedure is used to replace missing observations with values estimated from the rest of the data. For technical details readers are referred to Little and Rubin (1987) and Heyting *et al.* (1992). The approach can be illustrated using the HRT data, where the maximum likelihood estimates of the missing values are shown in Table 6.12. These values could now be used in any of the analyses discussed earlier, so that all forty patients could be included. This is left as an exercise for the reader. It should be noted however, that analysing 'filled-in' data as if they were complete, is likely to lead to overstatement of precision, that is standard errors are underestimated, stated *p*-values of tests are too small, and confidence intervals do not cover the true parameter at the stated rate.

Table 6.12 Maximum likelihood estimates of missing values in HRT study

Patient 5: Visit 3 = 3.86, Visit 4 = 5.60
Patient 13: Visit 4 = 5.84
Patient 16: Visit 3 = 5.09, Visit 4 = 6.23
Patient 25: Visit 4 = 3.58

(Software for handling missing data in longitudinal studies is available, notably the BMDP program, 5V.)

6.4 Analysis of covariance

Analysis of covariance is essentially analysis of variance in which differences between groups are tested, *after controlling for other variables*, termed covariates. The response variable and the covariate are assumed to be related in some way and from the estimated relationship, the subject's response scores are adjusted in an attempt to account for group differences in the covariates. Following this adjustment, the usual analysis-of-variance tests are applied to assess whether groups differ with respect to the response variable. To illustrate the techniques the data in Table 6.13 will be used. These data are anxiety scores of patients attending a hospital for wisdom tooth extraction. Scores are given before the operation and on discharge using the Spielberger anxiety inventory. Subjects were randomly allocated to one of three different methods of extraction. The main interest here is in group differences in anxiety on discharge, *controlling* for initial anxiety.

The analysis of covariance model assumes that anxiety on discharge and initial anxiety are linearly related and that the slope of the regression line is the same in each group. Specifically the model has the form

$$y_{ij} = \mu + \alpha_i + \beta(x_{ij} - \bar{x}_{..}) + \epsilon_{ij} \qquad (6.17)$$

where y_{ij} is the value of the response variable for the jth subject in the ith group and x_{ij} is the corresponding covariate value. Other terms in the model are

μ = overall mean,
α_i = effect of ith group ($i = 1, 2, 3, 4$),
β = slope of line,
ϵ_{ij} = residual or error term.

Estimates of group effects, error variation and between-group variation are all adjusted for the assumed relationship between dependent variable and covariate. Estimated group effects, for example, become

$$\hat{\alpha}_i = (\bar{y}_{i.} - \bar{y}_{..}) - \hat{\beta}(\bar{x}_{i.} - \bar{x}_{..}) \qquad (6.18)$$

rather than simply

$$\hat{\alpha}_i = (\bar{y}_{i.} - \bar{y}_{..}) \qquad (6.19)$$

where $\hat{\beta}$ is the least squares estimate of the slope of the regression line. An

Table 6.13 Anxiety scores for patients undergoing wisdom tooth extraction by one of three methods

Patient	Age (yrs)	Initial anxiety	Anxiety on discharge
Method 1			
1	27	30.2	32.0
2	32	35.3	34.8
3	23	32.4	36.0
4	28	31.9	34.2
5	30	28.4	30.3
6	35	30.5	33.2
7	32	34.8	35.0
8	21	32.5	34.0
9	26	33.0	34.2
10	27	29.9	31.1
Method 2			
11	29	32.6	31.5
12	29	33.0	32.9
13	31	31.7	34.3
14	36	34.0	32.8
15	23	29.9	32.5
16	26	32.2	32.9
17	22	31.0	33.1
18	20	32.0	30.4
19	28	33.0	32.6
20	32	31.1	32.8
Method 3			
21	33	29.9	34.1
22	35	30.0	34.1
23	21	29.0	33.2
24	28	30.0	33.0
25	27	30.0	34.1
26	23	29.6	31.0
27	25	32.0	34.0
28	26	31.0	34.0
29	27	30.1	35.0
30	29	31.0	36.0

estimate of error variation is obtained by subtracting that portion of the within-group sum-of-squares that is due to the covariance of x_{ij} and y_{ij}.

Returning now to the anxiety data, Table 6.14, shows the results of a simple one-way analysis of variance of anxiety on discharge and Table 6.15 the corresponding analysis of covariance using initial anxiety as a covariate. The results in Table 6.14 indicate that there is no difference in mean anxiety in the three method groups, but those in Table 6.15 suggest that after allowing for initial anxiety values, that the methods *do* differ on discharge anxiety means. The mean for each method, *adjusted* for initial values are also shown in Table 6.15, and show that anxiety scores on discharge are higher for method three than for the other two methods. (Adjusted estimates such as these must, of course, be interpreted with caution since their values depend heavily on the assumptions of linearity and equal slope.)

Table 6.14 One way analysis-of-variance results for anxiety on discharge – Table 6.13

Source	d.f.	Mean square	F	p
Between methods	2	4.32	2.13	0.14
Within methods	27	2.02		

Table 6.15 Analysis of covariance for anxiety on discharge using initial anxiety as covariate – Data in Table 6.13

Source	d.f.	Mean square	F	p
Initial anxiety	1	18.44	13.23	0.001
Between methods	2	10.12	7.26	0.003
Within methods	26	1.39		

Estimate of regression coefficient 0.54
Adjusted cell means for anxiety on discharge
  Method 1 33.21
  Method 2 32.22
  Method 3 34.48

The model in (6.17) may be extended in a straightforward manner to situations where the investigator wishes to allow for more than a single covariate. In the tooth extraction study, for example, it may be of interest to introduce age of patient in addition to initial anxiety value as a covariate when analysing anxiety scores on discharge. The new analysis of covariance results are shown in Table 6.16.

Analysis of covariance may also be used in association with repeated measure designs. To illustrate, the HRT study data of Table 6.7 will be used. One possible analysis is to use the mean of the four post-treatment values as the response and the mean of the two pre-treatment values as covariate. The results of such an analysis are given in Table 6.17. With this analysis no significant between group difference is found. The post-treatment difference between the two groups appears to be explicable in terms of the pre-treatment difference.

Frison and Pocock (1992) examine in detail the differences between the possible summary measure analyses of repeat measure designs, namely using post-treatment means only, using change scores and analysis of covariance of post-treatment mean with pre-treatment mean as covariate. A useful way of illustrating the differences is to look at the sample sizes required by each approach to detect a difference of a particular size with a specified power. (The required formulae, which assume equal correlations between the repeated measures, are given in Frison and Pocock.) Figure 6.4 illustrates results obtained for a situation involving four post-treatment measures and a single pre-treatment value, with an assumed correlation of 0.7. To obtain a power of 80%, analysis-of-covariance requires about 18 subjects per group, analysis of change scores about 24 and analysis of post-treatment scores only, about

Table 6.16   Analysis of covariance for anxiety on discharge using initial anxiety and age as covariates – Table 6.13

Source	d.f.	Mean square	F	p
Initial anxiety	1	16.88	11.74	0.002
Age	1	0.30	0.21	0.652
Between methods	2	9.89	6.88	0.004
Within methods	25	1.44		

Estimates of regression coefficients: initial anxiety 0.53
Age   0.02
Adjusted cell means for anxiety on discharge
Method 1 33.21
Method 2 32.24
Method 3 34.47

Table 6.17   Analysis of covariance of mean post-treatment HRT scores with mean pre-treatment as covariate

Source	SS	d.f.	MS	F	p
Groups	2.04	1	2.04	2.57	0.1184
Error	26.27	33	0.80		

50. Clearly for repeated measures which are moderately correlated, analysis of covariance is far more efficient than both the competing methods.

The analysis of covariance was first introduced by Fisher (1932) and was originally intended to be used in investigations where randomization had been used to assign patients to treatment groups. Experimental precision could be increased by removing from the error term that part of the residual variability in the response, linearly predictable from the covariate. Gradually however the technique has become more widely used to test hypotheses which are generally stated in such terms as 'the mean group differences on the response are zero when the group means on the covariate are made equal', or 'the group means on the response after adjustment for mean differences on the covariate are equal'. Indeed some authors, for example, McNemar (1962) have suggested that 'if there is only a small chance difference between the groups on the covariate, the use of covariance adjustment may not be worth the effort'. Such a comment rules out the situation for which the analysis of covariance was originally intended, since in the case of randomization, any group differences on the covariate are necessarily the result of chance. Such advice is clearly unsound because when analysis of covariance is used in association with random allocation, more powerful tests of group differences result because of the decrease in experimental error achieved.

In fact, it is where analysis of covariance is used in an attempt to undo built-in differences among intact groups that causes concern. Figure 6.5, for example, shows a plot of reaction time and age for psychiatric patients belonging to two distinct diagnostic groups. An analysis of covariance with reaction time as

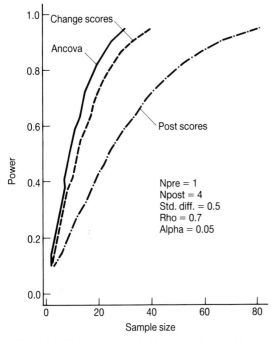

Figure 6.4 Power curves for three possible methods of analysing repeated measure designs

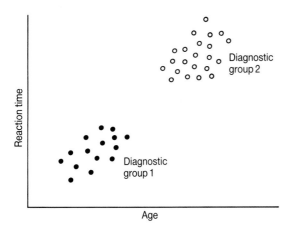

Figure 6.5 Plot of reaction time against age for two groups of psychiatric patients

response and age as covariate might here lead to the conclusion that reaction time does not differ in the two groups. In other words, given that two patients, one from each group, are of approximately the same age, then the reaction times are also likely to be similar. Is such a conclusion sensible? Examination of Figure 6.5 clearly shows that it is not, since the ages of the two groups do not overlap and analysis of covariance has essentially extrapolated into a region with no data. It is presumably this type of problem that caused Anderson (1963) to comment 'one may well wonder what exactly it means to ask what the data would be like if they weren't like they are'! Clearly some thought needs to be given to the use of analysis of covariance on intact groups and readers are referred to Fleiss and Tanur (1972) for more details.

6.5 Summary

Crossover designs, repeated measure studies and the analysis of covariance occur frequently in medical research. The 2×2 crossover design is appealing because by concentrating on within-subject constraints it promises more precise estimates of treatment effects for a given number of subjects. There are however a number of problems associated with the use of the design in practice, the most difficult of which is the assessment of possible carryover effects. Baseline measurements taken during a run-in and a washout period can be helpful in deriving unbiased estimates of treatment effects.

Longitudinal studies can be analysed in a variety of ways from the simple to the complex. The use of appropriate summary measures has a number of advantages. Baseline measurements can often be used as covariates in an analysis of covariance to provide more sensitive tests of treatment effects. Drop-outs in longitudinal studies are all too frequent a problem. All suggested approaches have their problems but imputing values for those missing using a maximum likelihood approach, may be the most satisfactory in many circumstances.

7

The Analysis of Survival Data

7.1 Introduction

In many medical investigations the most important response variable often involves time. Time from start of treatment to the first response, tumour-free time and length of remission are examples. Although in almost all such cases the observations are referred to as *survival times*, the endpoint of interest is not necessarily the death of a patient; it could be withdrawal because of severe side effects, the development of a tumour or numerous other events. Questions of interest for such data involve comparisons of survival times for different groups of patients, treated and untreated for example, and the identification of prognostic factors important for predicting survival times. These are similar questions to those that were of concern in earlier chapters and the question therefore arises as to why survival times merit special consideration. There are two main reasons. The first is that the distribution of survival times is often markedly skew or far from normality in some other way. (A set of data used in Chapter 5 illustrates this point.) The second, and perhaps more important reason, is the presence of *censored observations*. These arise because, at the completion of the study, some patients may not have reached the endpoint of interest (death, relapse, etc.). Consequently their exact survival times are not known. All that *is* known is that the survival times are *greater* than the amount of time the patient has been in the study. Censored observations may also occur when patients are lost to follow-up for any reason. These particular features mean that survival data generally require special methods of analysis and it is these which are the subject of this chapter.

7.2 The survival function and hazard function

Of central importance in the analysis of survival data are two functions describing the distribution of survival times, the *survival function* and the *hazard function*.

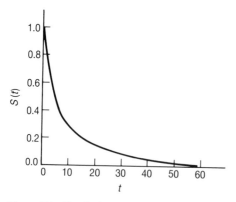

Figure 7.1   Survival curve

7.2.1 The survival function

Using T to represent survival time, this function, usually denoted by $S(t)$, is defined as the probability that an individual survives longer than t.

$$S(t) = P(T > t) \tag{7.1}$$

From the definition of the cumulative distribution function, $F(t)$, of T, as

$$F(t) = P(T < t) \tag{7.2}$$

it is seen that $S(t)$ may be written as

$$S(t) = 1 - F(t) \tag{7.3}$$

The graph of $S(t)$ against t is known as the *survival curve*. Two examples of such curves are shown in Figures 7.1 and 7.2. The gradual decline of the second curve indicates longer survival times, than for the steeper curve in Figure 7.1.

Estimation of the survival function and the construction of survival curves from observed survival times is discussed in Section 7.3.

7.2.2 The hazard function

In the analysis of survival data it is often of great interest to assess which periods have the highest and lowest chance of death, (or whatever the event of interest happens to be), *amongst those alive at the time*. In the very old, for example, there is a high risk of dying each year *among* those entering that stage of their life. The probability of any individual dying, say, in the 100th year is small because so few individuals live to be 100 years old. The appropriate device for assessing such risks is the *hazard function*, $h(t)$, which is defined as the probability that an individual experiences an event (death, relapse, etc.), in a small time interval, s, given that the individual has survived up to the beginning of this interval. In mathematical terms,

$$h(t) = \lim_{s \to 0} \frac{P(\text{event in } t, t + s)}{s} \tag{7.4}$$

The hazard function is also known as the *instantaneous failure rate* and the *age-specific failure rate*. It is a measure of how likely an individual is to experience

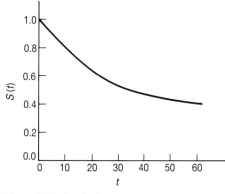

Figure 7.2 Survival curve

an event as a function of the age of the individual. The hazard function may remain constant, increase, decrease or take on some more complex shape. The hazard function for death in human beings, for example, has the shape shown in Figure 7.3. It is relatively high immediately after birth, declines rapidly in the early years and then remains approximately constant before beginning to rise again during late middle age.

The hazard function can also be defined in terms of the cumulative distribution function, $F(t)$, and the probability density function of the survival times, $f(t)$, as

$$h(t) = \frac{f(t)}{1 - F(t)} \tag{7.5}$$

The hazard function is also related to the survivor function by the relationship

$$S(t) = \exp(-\int_0^t h(x)dx) \tag{7.6}$$

The integral term in 7.6 is known as the *integrated hazard* and is important in particular analyses of survival data.

The hazard function can be estimated as the proportion of individuals experiencing an event in an interval per unit time, given that they have survived to the beginning of the interval, that is

$$\hat{h}(t) =$$

$$\frac{\text{number of individuals experiencing an event in the interval beginning at time } t}{(\text{number of patients surviving at } t) \; (\text{interval width})} \tag{7.7}$$

7.3 Estimating and testing the survival function

Table 7.1 shows the survival times in weeks of 20 stage 3 and 4 melanoma patients. Here there are no censored observations since all patients were followed up until they died. The survival function for any value of t is

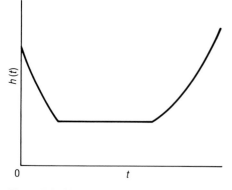

Figure 7.3   Hazard function for death in human beings

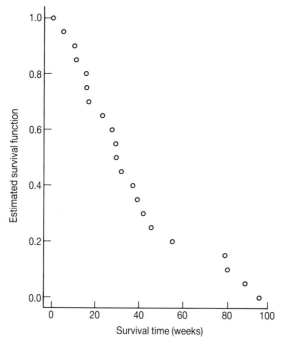

Figure 7.4   Estimated survival curve for the data in Table 7.1

estimated simply as the proportion of patients surviving longer than t,

$$\hat{S}(t) = \frac{\text{number of patients surviving longer than } t}{\text{total number of patients}} \tag{7.8}$$

Since every patient is alive at the beginning of the study and no-one is observed to survive longer than the largest of the observed survival times then,

$$\hat{S}(0) = 1 \text{ and } \hat{S}(t_{\max}) = 0 \tag{7.9}$$

Table 7.1 Ordered survival times for 20 patients with stage 3 and 4 melanoma

Survival time (weeks)	$\hat{S}(t)$
4.8	0.95
10.0	0.90
10.8	0.85
15.6	0.80
15.8	0.75
16.8	0.70
23.2	0.65
27.6	0.60
29.2	0.55
29.6	0.50
32.0	0.45
37.2	0.40
39.2	0.35
42.0	0.30
45.6	0.25
55.2	0.20
78.7	0.15
80.0	0.10
88.0	0.05
94.4	0.00

The estimated survival function for the melanoma patients is also shown in Table 7.1 and the corresponding survival curve appears in Figure 7.4. From this figure quantities like the median survival time might be found; here the value of t corresponding to $\hat{S}(t) = 0.5$ is 29.6 weeks.

The simple method of estimating the survival function described above can only be used if all individuals are followed up until the particular event of interest (in this example, death), has happened to each. In most survival time data sets however, there will be a number of censored observations, and an alternate procedure for estimating the survival function becomes necessary. Table 7.2, for example, shows further survival time data for stage 3 and 4 melanoma patients; here a number of patients are still alive at the end of the study.

To estimate the survival function for data containing censored observations, the most usual method is that described by Kaplan and Meier (1958), and known generally as the *product limit estimator*. The essence of the procedure is the use of the continued product of a series of conditional probabilities. For example, if it was required to find the probability of surviving say two years in a particular study, the following could be used

$$P(\text{surviving two years}) \quad = \quad P(\text{surviving one year}) \times P(\text{surviving two years}|$$
$$\text{having survived one year}) \qquad (7.10)$$

and the probability of surviving three years

$$P(3) = P(3|2) \times P(2) = P(3|2) \times P(2|1) \times P(1) \qquad (7.11)$$

Table 7.2 Ordered survival times for 20 patients with stage 3 and 4 melanoma and status of patients at end of the study

Survival time (weeks)	Status
12.8	dead
15.6	dead
24.0	alive
26.4	dead
29.2	dead
30.8	alive
39.2	dead
42.0	dead
58.4	alive
72.0	alive
77.2	dead
82.4	dead
87.2	alive
94.4	alive
97.2	alive
106.0	alive
114.8	alive
117.2	alive
140.0	alive
168.0	alive

In this way censored observation can be accommodated correctly.

The method is most easily explained by means of an example. Here the data in Table 7.2 will be used.

(1) $\hat{S}(12.8)$ = Proportion of patients surviving longer than 12.8 weeks
$\hat{S}(12.8)$ = $19/20 = 0.95 = P_1$(say),

(2) $\hat{S}(15.6)$ = $P_1 \times$ Proportion of patients surviving longer than 15.6 weeks given they have survived up to 15.6 weeks.
$\hat{S}(15.6)$ = $P_1 \times 18/19 = 19/20 \times 18/19 = 0.90 = P_2$

Up to this point the estimates are identical to those given by the method described earlier since there are no intervening censored observations. The estimate for the next time point, however, has to take account of the elimination of the observation censored at 24 weeks from the patients at risk at 26.4 weeks.

(3) $\hat{S}(26.4)$ = $P_1 \times P_2 \times$ Proportion of patients surviving longer than 26.4 weeks given that they have survived up to 26.4 weeks.
$\hat{S}(26.4)$ = $P_1 \times P_2 \times 16/17 = 0.847$ etc.

These calculations lead to the estimated survival curve for the data in Table 7.2 shown in Figure 7.5. The censored observations in these data are indicated by 'ticks' in Figure 7.5.

In general the product moment estimator of the survival curve involves

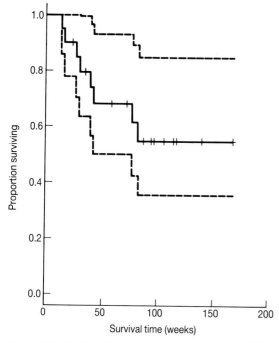

Figure 7.5 Kaplan–Meier survival curve for data in Table 7.2 showing 95% confidence interval

ordering the survival times from smallest to largest such that

$$t_{(1)} \leqslant t_{(2)} \ldots \leqslant t_{(n)} \tag{7.12}$$

and then finding the survivor function from

$$\hat{S}(t) = \prod_{t_{(r)} \leqslant t} \left(1 - \frac{d_j}{r_j} \right) \tag{7.13}$$

where r_j is the number of individuals at risk at t_j, and d_j is the number who experience the event of interest at t_j. (Individuals censored at t_j are included in r_j).

The variance of the Kaplan–Meier estimator can be estimated from

$$\text{var}(\hat{S}(t)) = [\hat{S}(t)]^2 \sum_{t_{(r)} \leqslant t} \frac{d_j}{r_j(r_j - d_j)} \tag{7.14}$$

Use of the general formula in (7.13) is illustrated on the data in Table 7.2 in Table 7.3. The 95% confidence interval for the survival curve, calculated using 7.14, is shown in Figure 7.5 by the two dash lines.

7.3.1 Comparing survival curves

Although the survival function of a single group of patients is a useful description of their survival times, it is often the comparison of the survival functions

Table 7.3 Estimating the survival curve and its standard error for the data in Table 7.2

t_j	r_j	d_j	$1-\frac{d_j}{r_j}$	$\hat{S}(t)$	SE	LCI	UCI
12.8	20	1	0.9500	0.9500	0.0487	0.8591	1.0000
15.6	19	1	0.9474	0.9003	0.0671	0.7777	1.0000
26.4	17	1	0.9412	0.8474	0.0814	0.7017	1.0000
29.2	16	1	0.9375	0.7944	0.0919	0.6329	0.9963
39.2	14	1	0.9286	0.7377	0.1013	0.5632	0.9654
42.0	13	1	0.9231	0.6810	0.1082	0.4983	0.9300
77.2	10	1	0.9000	0.6129	0.1169	0.4214	0.8904
82.4	9	1	0.8889	0.5448	0.1221	0.3508	0.8452

LCI = lower end of 95% confidence interval
UCI = upper end of 95% confidence interval

Table 7.4 Survival times for males and females

Patient	Sex	Survival time (weeks)	Status at end of study
1	M	2.3	Dead
2	M	4.8	Alive
3	M	6.1	Dead
4	M	15.2	Dead
5	M	23.8	Alive
6	F	1.6	Dead
7	F	3.8	Dead
8	F	14.3	Alive
9	F	18.7	Dead
10	F	36.3	Alive

of different groups of patients which is of greater interest. A clinician may, for example, wish to compare the survival times of males and females afflicted with some particular complaint. A medical researcher may wish to compare the retinopathy-free times of two groups of diabetic patients. In a clinical trial survival times of patients given an active treatment may need to be compared with those given a placebo.

Examples of data sets for which a comparison of survival curves is required are shown in Table 7.4 and 7.5. For the data in Table 7.4, for example, what is needed is a formal test of the hypothesis

$$H_0 : S_m = S_f \qquad (7.15)$$

where S_m and S_f are the survival functions of males and females.

In the absence of censored observations, standard non-parametric tests might be used to compare the survival times of each group (or even a two-sample t test if the distributions were approximately normal). When the data do contain censored observations there are a number of modified tests, both parametric and nonparametric, which may be used to compare the survival times. Here only the latter will be discussed.

Table 7.5 Initial remission times (days) for leukaemia patients

---

Treatment 1
4,5,9,10,11,12,13,23,28,28,28,29,31,32,37,41,41,57,62,74,100,139,20+,258+,269+
Treatment 2
8,10,10,12,14,20,48,70,75,99,103,162,169,195,220,161+,199+,217+,245+
Treatment 3
8,10,11,23,25,25,28,28,31,31,40,48,89,124,143,12+,159+,190+,196+,197+,205+,219+

'+' denotes a censored observation

Four nonparametric tests for assessing the equality of survival curves are available. Although the tests perform differently in some situations, their results will usually agree. They all have a normal approximation with associated probability levels, but these should be used with caution because they are strictly only applicable for large sample sizes. The four tests are as follows.

(1) *Peto/Wilcoxon* : a generalization of Wilcoxon's two-sample rank-sum test. This test and Gehan's Wilcoxon test (see below) have more power than the other tests when the hazard ratio is constant across time and the data are from the Weibull distribution (see Lee, 1991).

(2) *Gehan's Wilcoxon*: a generalization of Wilcoxon's two-sample rank-sum test (Gehan, 1965).

(3) *Log-Rank or Mantel–Haenszel Test*: Compares the observed number of deaths occurring at each particular time point with the number to be expected if the survival experience of the two groups is the same.

(4) *Cox–Mantel Test*: this test is similar to the log-rank test. (Cox, 1959, 1972, Mantel, 1966).

All of these tests are illustrated in Lee (1991). Here a brief account of the log-rank test will be given, using first the small set of data shown in Table 7.4. A 2×2 table giving the number of individuals dying and the number remaining alive *and* at risk is constructed for the different times at which deaths occur. These tables, for the data in Table 7.4, are shown in Table 7.6. Assuming the probability of death is the same for males and females, the relevant expected values for each table can be calculated from the appropriate row and column marginal totals in the usual way as when testing for independence.The observed and expected values for each group at each time point are then summed to give the values also shown in Table 7.6. These values can be compared by a simple approximate statistic given by

$$X^2 = \frac{(O_f - E_f)^2}{E_f} + \frac{(O_m - E_m)^2}{E_m} \qquad (7.16)$$

leading in this case to the value 0.008. Under the null hypothesis of equal survival curves for males and females the statistic in (7.16) has, approximately, a chi-square distribution with a single degree of freedom. Here there is no evidence of a difference in the survival experience of men and women.

The log-rank test is not restricted to the two-group situation and can be used to assess the equality of survival curves from any number of groups. As

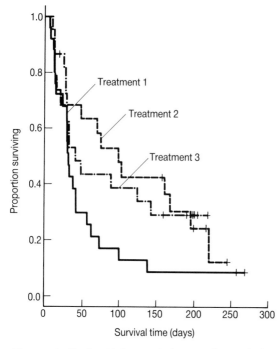

Figure 7.6   Kaplan–Meier survival curves for remission times of leukaemia patients in three treatment groups (Table 7.5)

an example consider the data shown in Table 7.5 taken from Lee (1991). These data involve initial remission times of leukaemia patients induced by three treatments. Here the observed and expected number of deaths in the three groups calculated as described above are

Group	Observed	Expected
1	22	15.37
2	15	18.69
3	15	17.94

The resulting test statistic takes the value 4.3. In this case, where three groups are involved, this is tested as a chi-square with two degrees of freedom. The resulting p value is 0.1137 suggesting that there is no difference between the three treatments. The Kaplan–Meier survival curves for the three groups are shown in Figure 7.6.

Table 7.6 Calculation of log-rank test for data in Table 7.4

Time		M	F	Total
1.6		*M*	*F*	*Total*
	Dead	0(0.5)	1(0.5)	1
	Alive	5	4	9
	Total	5	5	10
2.3		*M*	*F*	*Total*
	Dead	1(0.55)	0(0.45)	1
	Alive	4	4	8
	Total	5	4	9
3.8		*M*	*F*	*Total*
	Dead	0(0.5)	1(0.5)	1
	Alive	4	3	7
	Total	4	4	8
6.1		*M*	*F*	*Total*
	Dead	1(0.5)	0(0.5)	1
	Alive	2	3	5
	Total	3	3	6
15.2		*M*	*F*	*Total*
	Dead	1(0.5)	0(0.5)	1
	Alive	1	2	3
	Total	2	2	4
18.7		*M*	*F*	*Total*
	Dead	0(0.33)	1(0.67)	1
	Alive	1	1	2
	Total	1	2	3

Expected number of deaths are shown in parentheses. 'Alive' means alive *and* at risk
Observed number of deaths for men = 3
Expected number of deaths for men = 0.5 + 0.56 + 0.5 + 0.5 + 0.5 + 0.33 = 2.89
Observed number of deaths for women = 3
Expected number of deaths for women = 0.5 + 0.44 + 0.5 + 0.5 + 0.5 + 0.67 = 3.11

7.4 The effect of prognostic factors on survival time

In several earlier chapters it was seen that one of the main aims of many medical investigations is the identification of prognostic factors related to the response variable of interest. This remains true in studies involving survival times. Because of the special features of such data, however, the straightforward multiple regression approach described in Chapter 5 is not appropriate. A number of more suitable models have now been developed, of which perhaps the most successful is that due to Cox (1972). Most such models are centred around the hazard function, since this is a simpler vehicle for modelling the joint effects of prognostic variables than the survival function, since it does not involve the cumulative history of events. To introduce the basic concepts suppose firstly that only two explanatory variables, x_1 and x_2, are of interest and that these do not vary with time. A first step in the modelling process might be to assume that $h(t)$ is a linear function of x_1 and x_2. Such a model is, however, not really suitable since $h(t)$ is restricted to being positive, whereas the postulated linear function would not necessarily be likewise constrained (compare Chapter 5 and the discussion of logistic regression). A more sensible model is one that involves a linear model for the logarithm of the hazard function, that is

$$\ln h(t) = \beta_0 + \beta_1 x_1 + \beta_2 x_2 \qquad (7.17)$$

where β_0, β_1 and β_2 are parameters which will need to be estimated from observed data. In (7.17) the hazard function is modelled as depending on the two prognostic variables, x_1 and x_2, but *not* dependent on time. A hazard function which is constant over time arises only when the distribution of survival times is exponential, when (7.17) is referred to as an *exponential regression model*. Such a model is very restrictive since hazard functions which increase or decrease with time are much more likely. A suitable model in such cases would be

$$\ln h(t) = \beta_0 + \beta_1 x_1 + \beta_2 x_2 + \beta_3 t \qquad (7.18)$$

Depending on the sign of β_3, such a model could represent a hazard function increasing or decreasing with time.

The coefficients in models such as (7.17) and (7.18) can be estimated by maximum likelihood methods (see Allison, 1984, for details), and this might be useful in many situations. The models do, however, have a number of disadvantages. Firstly, it is necessary to decide how the hazard function depends on time and in general there may be little information available on which to base a choice. Secondly, if the hazard is believed to be *non-monotonic* (that is, it does not simply increase or decrease with time but varies in a more complex fashion), then it may be difficult to find an appropriate explicit function of time to include in the model. Such problems are overcome in the *proportional hazards model* suggested by Cox (1972). Essentially this involves a generalization of models such as (7.17) and (7.18) in which the dependence of $h(t)$ on t does not have to be specified explicitly. For the situation with two explanatory variables considered above, the model is

$$\ln h(t) = \ln \alpha(t) + \beta_0 + \beta_1 x_1 + \beta_2 x_2 \qquad (7.19)$$

where $\alpha(t)$, is any function of time. The term 'proportional hazards' arises because for any two individuals at any point in time, the model in (7.19) specifies that the ratio of their hazards is a constant. In other words, if an individual has a risk of death at some initial time point that is twice as high as another individual, then at all later times the risk of death remains twice as high. Proportionality of hazards is an assumption that may not necessarily hold. For example, if two individuals with a heart condition receive different treatments, one medical and one surgical, then the individual being treated surgically may be at higher risk initially because of the possibility of operative mortality. At a later stage, however, the risk may become the same or even less than for the medically treated individual. In this case, if one of the covariates is a dummy variable indicating whether a person is treated surgically or medically, then the proportional hazards model will not hold. (This example was suggested by Fisher and van Belle, 1993.) In a given situation the proportionality assumption needs to be checked (see later).

Nevertheless Cox's model has proved extremely useful and has become very popular since it was published.

It may be helpful to examine the model in (7.19) in a little more detail. For the general situation involving p covariates, the model may be rewritten as

$$h(t) = \alpha(t) \exp\left(\beta_0 + \sum_{i=1}^{p} \beta_i x_i \right) \qquad (7.20)$$

The baseline hazard function, $\alpha(t)$, corresponds to that for the average value of all the covariates (see Lee, 1991). For an individual with covariate values $\mathbf{x}' = [x_1, x_2, \ldots, x_p]$, the hazard function is $\alpha(t)C$ where C is a constant, the value of which depends on the values in $\mathbf{x}$ and the estimated coefficients in the model. For two individuals with covariate values $\mathbf{x}_1$ and $\mathbf{x}_2$ the ratio of the two hazard functions is

$$\frac{\alpha(t)C(\mathbf{x}_1)}{\alpha(t)C(\mathbf{x}_2)} = \frac{C(\mathbf{x}_1)}{C(\mathbf{x}_2)} \qquad (7.21)$$

The ratio does not depend on t.

Because the baseline hazard function, $\alpha(t)$, does not have to be specified explicitly, the proportional hazards model is essentially non-parametric. To estimate the parameters in the proportional hazards model Cox devised a *conditional likelihood* procedure, for details of which readers are referred to the original paper or to Chapter 4 of Kalbfleisch and Prentice (1980). The central idea of the estimation process however is that only the *order* in which events occur is of importance, not the exact times they occur.

To introduce the use of Cox's proportional hazards model it will be applied to the remission times of leukaemia patients given in Table 7.5. The times for the first two treatments will be used, with treatment group (0 = treatment 1, 1 = treatment 2), being used as a single covariate. The results are shown in Table 7.7. From the parameter estimates two 'conversion' factors can be calculated which are useful in interpreting and applying the results of the analysis. The calculation of these is also shown in Table 7.7. Using the relationship between the hazard function and survival function given in (7.6) the survival functions of the two treatments are seen to be

$$S_1(t) = [S_0(t)]^{C_1}, \; S_2(t) = [S_0(t)]^{C_2} \qquad (7.22)$$

where $S_0(t)$ is the baseline survival function corresponding to the baseline hazard, $\alpha(t)$. $S_0(t)$ can be estimated by a method given in Link (1984) and is again given in Table 7.7. From the estimated values of $S_0(t)$, (7.22) can be used to find the corresponding values for the two treatment groups. For example, the baseline survival estimate for ten weeks is 0.8299. Consequently the estimated ten weeks survival probability for patients in treatment group one is $0.8299^{1.323} = 0.7814$ and for those in treatment group two, $0.8299^{0.692} = 0.8790$.

As a further more complex example of the application Cox's model it will be applied to the data shown in Table 7.8 taken from Lee (1991). Fifty one previously untreated adult patients with acute myeloblastic leukaemia were given a course of treatment and their survival times recorded along with five pre-treatment variables

Table 7.7   Results of Cox's regression for remission times of leukaemia patients

Parameter estimates
$\hat{\beta}_0 = 0.2800$, $\hat{\beta}_1 = -0.6484$
Conversion factors
$C_1 = \exp(0.2800 - 0.6484 \times 0) = \exp(0.2800) = 1.323$
$C_2 = \exp(0.2800 - 0.6484 \times 1) = \exp(-0.3684) = 0.6918$
Estimated baseline survival

Survival time	Status	Baseline survival
4	D	0.9786
5	D	0.9570
8	D	0.9353
9	D	0.9138
10	D	0.8299
10	D	0.8299
10	D	0.8299
10	D	0.8299
12	D	0.7869
12	D	0.7869
13	D	0.7650
14	D	0.7430
20	D	0.7211
20	C	0.7211
23	D	0.6986
28	D	0.6324
28	D	0.6324
28	D	0.6324
29	D	0.6088
31	D	0.5848
32	D	0.5604
37	D	0.5358
41	D	0.4869
41	D	0.4869
48	D	0.4609
57	D	0.4354
62	D	0.4094
70	D	0.3829
74	D	0.3569
75	D	0.3303
99	D	0.3043
100	D	0.2790
103	D	0.2529
139	D	0.2277
161	C	0.2004
162	D	0.1992
169	D	0.1720
195	D	0.1460
199	C	0.1403
217	C	0.1173
220	D	0.1139
245	C	-
258	C	-
269	C	-

D = dead
C = censored

Table 7.8 Data for 51 leukaemia patients

			Variable			
1	2	3	4	5	6	7
20	78	39	7	990	18	0
25	64	61	16	1030	31	1
26	61	55	12	982	31	0
26	64	64	16	1000	31	0
27	95	95	6	980	36	0
27	80	64	8	1010	1	0
28	88	88	20	986	9	0
28	70	70	14	1010	39	1
31	72	72	5	988	20	1
33	58	58	7	986	4	0
33	92	92	5	980	45	1
33	42	38	12	984	36	0
34	26	26	7	982	12	0
36	55	55	14	986	8	0
37	71	71	15	1020	1	0
40	91	91	9	986	15	0
40	52	49	12	988	24	0
43	74	63	4	986	2	0
45	78	47	14	980	33	0
45	60	36	10	992	29	1
45	82	32	10	1016	7	0
45	79	79	4	1030	0	0
47	56	28	2	990	1	0
48	60	54	10	1002	2	0
50	83	66	19	996	12	0
50	36	32	14	992	9	0
51	88	70	8	982	1	0
52	87	87	7	986	1	0
53	75	68	13	980	9	0
53	65	65	6	982	5	0
56	97	92	10	992	27	1
57	87	83	19	1020	1	0
59	45	45	8	999	13	0
59	36	34	5	1038	1	0
60	39	33	7	988	5	0
60	76	53	12	982	1	0
61	46	37	4	1006	3	0
61	39	8	8	990	4	0
61	90	90	11	990	1	0
62	84	84	19	1020	18	0
63	42	27	5	1014	1	0
65	75	75	10	1004	2	0
71	44	22	6	990	1	0
71	63	63	11	986	8	0
73	33	33	4	1010	3	0
73	93	84	6	1020	4	0
74	58	58	10	1002	14	0
74	32	30	16	988	3	0
75	60	60	17	990	13	0
77	69	69	9	986	13	0
80	73	73	7	986	1	0

Variables:
1 = Age at diagnosis
2 = Smear differential percentage of blasts
3 = Percentage of absolute marrow leukaemia infiltrate
4 = Percentage labelling index of the bone marrow leukaemia cells
5 = Highest temperature prior to treatment (degrees F; decimal points omitted)
6 = Survival time from diagnosis (months)
7 = Status (0 = dead, 1 = still alive)

(1)   Age at diagnosis (AGE),
(2)   Smear differential percentage of blasts (SMEAR),
(3)   Percentage of absolute marrow leukaemia infiltrate (INFIL)
(4)   Percentage labelling index of the bone marrow leukaemia cells (CELLS)
(5)   Highest temperature prior to treatment (TEMP).

A number of censored observations arose from those patients still alive at the end of the study period.

The estimates of the regression coefficients for each explanatory variable for Cox's model are shown in Table 7.9 along with their standard errors. Comparing each coefficient with the appropriate standard error appears to indicate that age alone is an important prognostic variable for survival time. For the moment however, a model including all five covariates will used. Once again, estimated survival values for individuals with a paticular pattern of covariate values can be found by applying the appropriate conversion factor to the estimated values of the baseline survival function. Consider, for example, an individual with the following five values, AGE = 50, SMEAR = 80, INFIL = 50, CELLS = 5, TEMP = 1030. The conversion factor for this patient is calculated as

$$
\begin{aligned}
C &= \exp(-14.81 + 0.0317 \times 50 + 0.0093 \times 80 - 0.0161 \\
&\quad \times 50 - 0.0592 \times 5 + 0.0142 \times 1030) \\
&= \exp(1.044) = 2.841
\end{aligned}
\tag{7.23}
$$

Consequently, for this individual the estimated chance of surviving more than 12 months is $0.3903^{2.841} = 0.0690$, since the estimated baseline 12 months survival is 0.3903.

As with the regression methods described in Chapter 5, important subsets of covariates in a Cox's regression model, can be chosen by a stepwise procedure, although the selection criterion used is different. Here such a procedure chooses AGE as the only significant prognostic variable. The new model which includes only AGE gives the estimate of the regression coefficient as 0.0311, with a standard error of 0.009 55. The corresponding z value is 3.25 with $p = 0.001\ 15$. Further interpretation of the estimated regression coefficients proceeds in the same way as for the unstandardized coefficients in multiple regression, so that, in this example, each additional year of life increases the logarithm of the hazard function by 0.0311. A more appealing interpretation is achieved by first exponentiating the coefficient to give 1.03, implying that the hazard function of an individual aged $x + 1$ is 1.03 times the hazard function of an individual aged x. An additional aid to interpretation is to calculate

$$
100(\exp(\text{coefficient}) - 1)
\tag{7.24}
$$

This value will give the percentage change in the hazard function with each unit change in the prognostic variable. So here, yearly increases in age lead to a 3% increase in the hazard function. An approximate 95% confidence interval for this value, found by applying (7.24) to the values of the coefficient $\pm$ 2 standard errors, is (1%, 5%).

As with other regression models discussed in earlier chapters, the next stage in a complete analysis is to examine residual and diagnostic plots for evidence

Table 7.9 Estimates of coefficients of Cox's regression model fitted to data on 51 leukaemia patients

Variable	Coefficient	SE
AGE	0.0317	0.0102
SMEAR	0.0093	0.0142
INFIL	−0.0161	0.0124
CELLS	−0.0592	0.0382
TEMP	0.0142	0.0110

The constant is estimated as −14.81

of outliers, influential observations, etc. A variety of such plots are available for Cox's proportional hazards model, all of which are described in detail in Therneau *et al.* (1990). The three types of residual which are of most use in practice are:

(a) *Martingale*: useful in uncovering the correct functional form for a covariate,
(b) *Deviance*: useful in identifying poorly predicted subjects,
(c) *Schoenfeld*: useful for assessing whether or not the proportional hazards function is appropriate.

The mathematics behind these residuals is complex and will not be described here. To illustrate the possibilities however, Figure 7.7 shows the deviance residuals plotted against age. Only the residual corresponding to observation 22 appears unusual. This individual has a recorded survival time of zero.

7.5 Assessing the adequacy of the conditional hazards model and time-dependent covariates

The proportional hazards model assumes that for two different sets of covariate values, x_1 and x_2, the hazard functions are related as follows

$$\frac{h(t, x_1)}{h(t, x_2)} = \exp \beta'(x_1 - x_2) \tag{7.25}$$

The ratio of the two hazard functions does not depend on time. Such an assumption has been found to be reasonable in many situations, hence the great popularity of Cox's model. Circumstances may however occur where an investigator wishes to check that such proportionality of hazards does indeed hold, or whether some alternative model might be necessary. Suppose for example that there is some suspicion that males and females have nonproportional hazards, the hazard for males increasing more with time than that for females. If x_1 is a dummy variable representing gender, coded 0 for women and 1 for men, a possible model is

$$\ln h(t) = \ln \alpha(t) + \beta_0 + \beta_1 x_1 + \beta_2 x_1 t \tag{7.26}$$

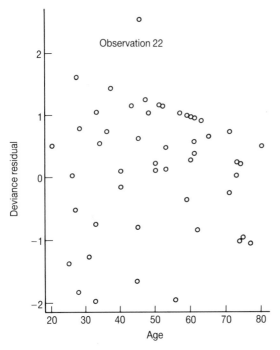

Figure 7.7   Deviance residuals for Cox's regression model with Age as covariate fitted to data on 51 leukaemia patients (Table 7.8)

If β_2 is positive than the model in (7.26) implies that the hazard for males increases more with time than that for females — $x_1 t$ is a *time-dependent* covariate. To test the proportionality of hazards assumption the parameters in (7.26) could be estimated and the hypothesis that $\beta_2 = 0$ tested. Other more complex interactions between covariates and time could be investigated in a similar fashion.

To illustrate this approach, part of the data given in Table 7.8 will be used. Age at diagnosis will again be used as a covariate along with temperature grouped into above and below 100°F. The new variable, *gtemp*, will be set to 0 for individuals with temperatures below 100°F and to 1 for individuals with temperatures of 100°F and above. The survival curves of the low and high temperature groups (see Figure 7.8), suggest that the survival experience of the latter group is different from that of the former, being initially worse but becoming better for longer survival times. A further indication that the proportionality of hazards assumption may not be valid for temperature group is seen in the plot of $\ln(-\ln \hat{S}_l(t))$ and $\ln(-\ln \hat{S}_h(t))$ against time, where $\hat{S}_l$ and $\hat{S}_h$ are estimates of the survival functions for the two temperature groups. This plot, seen in Figure 7.9, indicates that the differences in the two curves are *not* constant over time, whereas for proportionality to be valid, constant differences are required. (The rationale behind this type of plot is given in Kalbfleisch and Prentice, 1980.)

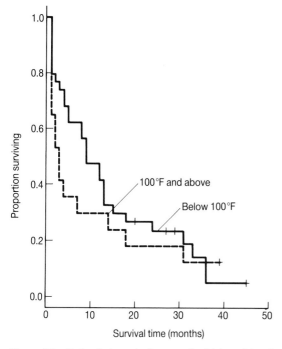

Figure 7.8 Estimated survival curves for high and low temperature groups

Table 7.10 Estimated coefficients in the model with temperature group fitted to data on leukaemia patients

Variable	Coefficient	SE
AGE	0.0314	0.0099
gtemp	0.7768	0.5128
Z	−1.0375	0.6957

Since there appears to be some evidence that temperature group may not meet the proportional hazards assumption, a Cox's regression with AGE, gtemp and a third covariate z was fitted where z was defined as

$$z = \text{gtemp} \times \ln(\text{survival time}) \qquad (7.27)$$

The estimated regression coefficients and their standard errors are shown in Table 7.10. Although the coefficient of z is not significantly different from zero, it is not entirely negligible and it may be that the proportionality of hazards assumption is not entirely satisfactory for temperature group.

A further more complex example involving time dependent covariates concerns the data collected in the Stanford heart transplant study (see Crowley and Hu, 1977). Survival information and observations on a number of covari-

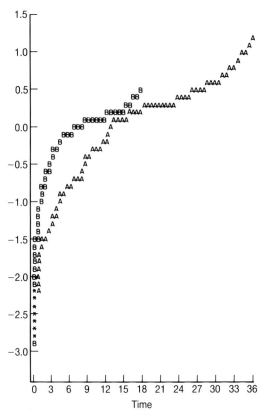

Figure 7.9   Log minus log plot for high and low temperature groups

ates were obtained for 99 patients accepted into the heart transplant program. The data are reproduced in Table 7.11. The variables recorded are:

(1) Patient identification,
(2) Survival time in days (TIME),
(3) Censoring status: incomplete = 0, complete = 1 (STATUS),
(4) Waiting time to transplant in days (WAIT),
(5) Age at transplant (AGE),
(6) tissue mismatch score (MISS).

Since here some patients received a heart transplant and others did not, information on all the covariates is not complete. The data will be used to illustrate how an event that possibly alters a patient's prognosis may be included in a Cox's regression as a time-dependent covariate. Three possibly informative covariates which depend upon the transplantation time will be investigated. The first, transplant status (TS) is a dummy variable equal to zero before transplantation and one afterwards. The second, age at transplant, is defined to be zero before transplant, as is the third, mismatch score. The

Table 7.11 Survival information and covariates for 99 patients accepted into a heart transplant programme

1	2	3	4	5	6
1	49	1			
2	5	1			
3	15	1	0	54	1.11
4	38	1	35	40	1.66
5	17	1			
6	2	1			
7	674	1	50	51	1.32
8	39	1			
9	84	1			
10	57	2	11	42	0.61
11	152	1	25	48	0.36
12	7	1			
13	80	1	16	54	1.89
14	1386	1	36	54	0.87
15	0	1			
16	307	1	27	49	1.12
17	35	1			
18	42	1	19	56	2.05
19	36	1			
20	27	1	17	55	2.76
21	1031	2	7	43	1.13
22	50	1	11	42	1.38
23	732	1	2	58	0.96
24	218	1	82	52	1.62
25	1799	0	24	33	1.06
26	1400	0			
27	262	1			
28	71	1	70	54	0.47
29	34	1			
30	851	1	15	44	1.58
31	15	1			
32	76	1	16	64	0.69
33	1586	0	50	49	0.91
34	1571	0	22	40	0.38
35	11	1			
36	99	1	45	49	2.09
37	65	1	18	61	0.87
38	4	1	4	41	0.87
40	1407	0	40	48	0.75
41	1321	0	57	45	0.98
42	2	1			
43	1	1			
44	39	1			
45	44	1	0	36	0.0
46	995	1	1	48	0.81
47	71	2	20	47	1.38
48	8	1			
49	1141	0	35	36	1.35
51	284	1	31	48	1.08
52	101	1			
54	2	1			
55	60	1	9	52	1.51

Table 7.11   *cont.*

1	2	3	4	5	6
56	941	0	66	38	0.98
57	148	1			
58	342	1	20	48	1.82
59	915	0	77	41	0.19
60	52	1	2	49	0.66
61	1	1			
62	68	1			
63	841	0	26	32	1.93
64	583	1	32	48	0.12
65	77	1	11	51	1.12
66	31	1			
67	284	1	56	19	1.02
68	67	1	2	45	1.68
69	669	0	9	48	1.20
70	29	1	4	53	1.68
71	619	0	30	47	0.97
72	595	0	3	26	1.46
73	89	1	26	56	2.16
74	16	1	4	29	0.61
75	1	1			
76	544	0	45	52	1.70
77	20	1			
78	514	0	209	49	0.81
79	95	1	66	54	1.08
80	481	0	25	46	1.41
81	444	0	5	52	1.94
82	427	0			
83	79	1	31	53	3.05
84	333	1	36	42	0.60
85		4	1		
86	396	0	7	48	1.44
87	109	1	59	46	2.25
88	369	0	30	54	0.68
89	206	1	138	51	1.33
90	185	1	159	52	0.82
91	339	1			
92	339	0	309	45	0.16
93	264	0	27	47	0.33
94	164	1	3	43	1.20
96	179	0	12	26	0.46
97	130	0	20	23	1.78
98	108	0	95	28	0.77
99	20	1			
100	38	0	37	35	0.67
101	30	0			
102	10	0			
103	5	1			

Variables:
1 = Patient identification
2 = TIME
3 = STATUS
4 = WAIT
5 = AGE
6 = MISS

Table 7.12 Estimated coefficients in the model fitted to heart transplant data

Variable	Coefficient	SE
TS	−3.6078	1.2694
AGE	0.0593	0.0242
MISS	0.5109	0.2924

estimated coefficients for these three covariates and their standard errors are shown in Table 7.12. Clearly being given a transplant decreases the hazard function, with the hazard function for those patients receiving a new heart being about 3% of that of patients not being transplanted. (An approximate 95% confidence interval is 0.0021, 0.34.) Increased age at transplant is associated with an increase in the hazard function as is a larger mismatch score. (For a more detailed account of the analysis of these data see Kalbfleisch and Prentice, 1980, and Cox and Oakes, 1984.)

7.6 Summary

Because of their non-normality and because of the presence of censored observations, survival time data require special techniques for their analysis. Survival curves can be compared by a variety of non-parametric techniques and the effects of prognostic variables on survival time can be assessed using Cox's proportional hazards model. Comprehensive accounts of the analysis of survival data are given in Kalbfleisch and Prentice (1980) Cox and Oakes (1984) and Lee (1991).

8

Reducing the Dimensionality of Multivariate Data: Principal Components Analysis, Factor Analysis and Correspondence Analysis

8.1 Introduction

In medical research, particularly in areas such as psychiatry and clinical psychology, investigations often involve the observation and recording of many variables on each of the individuals in the study. Table 8.1 for example, shows the values of five variables for each of ten individuals. There are a variety of questions that might be of interest for such *multivariate data*, but often the most important concerns are how to achieve a parsimonious description of the relationships and associations amongst the variables, and how to reduce the number of variables whilst preserving as much of the original information as possible. A technique which is particularly useful here is *principal components analysis,* but other methods such as *exploratory factor analysis* and *correspondence analysis* are also helpful in particular circumstances. Each of these will be described later in this chapter. Firstly, however, it will be useful to make some general comments about multivariate data. (Data sets discussed in previous chapters, for example, Chapters 5 and 7, which involved more than a single variable, are not considered multivariate since it is only the response that is assumed to be a random variable.)

8.2 Describing multivariate data

A set of multivariate data is generally represented by a matrix, $\mathbf{X}$, where

$$\mathbf{X} = \begin{pmatrix} x_{11} & x_{12} & \cdots & x_{1p} \\ x_{21} & x_{22} & \cdots & x_{2p} \\ \vdots & & & \vdots \\ x_{n1} & x_{n2} & \cdots & x_{np} \end{pmatrix} \qquad (8.1)$$

and n is the number of individuals or patients under investigation, p is the number of variables observed on each patient and x_{ij} represents the value of variable j for patient i.

Table 8.1   Hypothetical set of multivariate data

Individual	Sex	Age	IQ	Depressed?	Weight (lb)
1	male	21	120	yes	150
2	male	43	100	no	160
3	male	22	98	no	150
4	male	86	99	no	135
5	male	60	90	no	178
6	female	16	124	yes	120
7	female	20	112	no	131
8	female	43	95	yes	145
9	female	22	91	yes	167
10	female	80	101	yes	123

To summarize such data, sample means and variances could be calculated for each variable and sample covariances and correlations for each pair of variables. A convenient nomenclature for these summary statistics is shown in Table 8.2. In addition it may be useful to display the data graphically by plotting the scattergrams for each pair of variables, particularly if these are arranged in the form of a p by p grid — see below.

The use of the summary statistics detailed in Table 8.2 will be illustrated on the data set shown in Table 8.3. These data, taken from Neter *et al.* (1985) consist of muscle, skin and body fat measurements for 20 individuals. The results are shown in Table 8.4. Scatterplots of each pair of variables arranged in the form of a 4×4 grid are shown in Figure 8.1.

Often the number of variables in a set of multivariate data is quite large and the sheer volume of data can be be daunting. In such circumstances the researcher may want to reduce the number of variables in some way. One method would be simply to choose a subset of the original variables. In the body fat data, for example, tricep and thigh have a correlation of 0.92, so that it might be thought that only one of them is really needed in any analyses performed on the data. An alternative procedure is to construct a number of *new* variables from the p original variables. This may not be immediately so appealing as simply selecting a subset of the original variables, but it can have considerable advantages, as will be seen later. Particularly useful are derived variables which are *linear combinations* of the originals. Such a linear combination has the general form

$$y = a_1 x_1 + a_2 x_2 + \ldots + a_p x_p \tag{8.2}$$

where the as are a set of constants chosen so that the derived variable, y, has particular properties (see later). The mean, and more importantly the variance, of these linear combinations may be found from the means, variances and covariances of the original variables. Linear combinations such as (8.2) are the basis of principal components analysis which is now described in more detail.

Table 8.2 Summary statistics for multivariate data

(1) *Sample means*
Mean of *i*th variable, $\bar{x}_i = \frac{1}{n}\sum_{j=1}^{n} x_{ji}$
Vector of means of all p variables, $\bar{\mathbf{x}}' = [\bar{x}_1, \bar{x}_2, \ldots, \bar{x}_p]$.
(2) *Sample variances*
Sample variance of the *i*th variable, $s_{ii} = \frac{1}{n-1}\sum_{j=1}^{n}(x_{jj} - \bar{x}_i)^2$
(3) *Sample covariances*
Sample covariance between variables i and j, $s_{ij} = \frac{1}{n-1}\sum_{k=1}^{n}(x_{ki} - \bar{x}_i)(x_{kj} - \bar{x}_j)$
(4) *Sample covariance matrix*

$$\mathbf{S} = \begin{pmatrix} s_{11} & s_{12} & \cdots & s_{1p} \\ s_{21} & s_{22} & \cdots & s_{2p} \\ \vdots & \vdots & & \vdots \\ s_{p1} & s_{p2} & \cdots & s_{pp} \end{pmatrix}$$

(5) *Sample correlation*
Sample correlation between variables i and j, $r_{ij} = \frac{s_{ij}}{\sqrt{s_{ii}s_{jj}}}$
(6) *Sample correlation matrix*

$$\mathbf{R} = \begin{pmatrix} 1 & r_{12} & \cdots & r_{1p} \\ \vdots & & \vdots \\ r_{p1} & r_{p2} & \cdots & 1 \end{pmatrix}$$

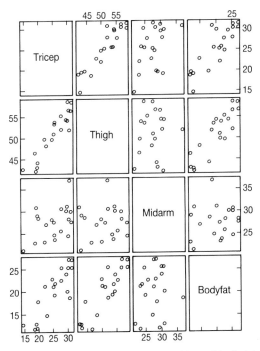

Figure 8.1 Scatterplots of muscle, skin and body fat measurements

Table 8.3   Muscle, skin and body fat measurements for 20 subjects

Variable			
1	2	3	4
19.5	43.1	29.1	11.9
24.7	49.8	28.2	22.8
30.7	51.9	37.0	18.7
29.8	54.3	31.1	20.1
19.1	42.2	30.9	12.9
25.6	53.9	23.7	21.7
31.4	58.5	27.6	27.1
27.9	52.1	30.6	25.4
22.1	49.9	23.2	21.3
25.5	53.5	24.8	19.3
31.1	56.6	30.0	25.4
30.4	56.7	28.3	27.2
18.7	46.5	23.0	11.7
19.7	44.2	28.6	17.8
14.6	42.7	21.3	12.8
29.5	54.4	30.1	23.9
27.7	55.3	25.7	22.6
30.2	58.6	24.6	25.4
22.7	48.2	27.1	14.8
25.2	51.0	27.5	21.1

1 Tricep — triceps skinfold thickness (mm)
2 Thigh — thigh circumference (cm)
3 Midarm — midarm circumference (cm)
4 Bodyfat — percent of body fat

Table 8.4   Summary statistics for muscle, skin and body fat data

1. *Sample means and variances*

	tricep	thigh	midarm	body fat
Mean	25.3	51.2	27.6	20.2
Variance	25.2	27.4	13.3	26.1

2. *Sample covariance matrix*

$$S = \begin{pmatrix} 25.2 & 24.3 & 8.4 & 21.6 \\ 24.3 & 27.4 & 1.6 & 23.5 \\ 8.4 & 1.6 & 13.3 & 2.7 \\ 21.6 & 23.5 & 2.7 & 26.1 \end{pmatrix}$$

3. *Sample correlation matrix*

$$R = \begin{pmatrix} 1.00 & 0.92 & 0.46 & 0.84 \\ 0.92 & 1.00 & 0.08 & 0.88 \\ 0.46 & 0.08 & 1.00 & 0.14 \\ 0.84 & 0.88 & 0.14 & 1.00 \end{pmatrix}$$

8.3 Principal components analysis

Principal components analysis is a method of data reduction which aims to produce a small number of derived variables that can be used in place of the larger number of original variables in subsequent analyses of the data. The new variables are defined to be linear combinations of the original variables, with the coefficients chosen so that the derived variables (the principal components) are uncorrelated and, in addition, are such that the first few of the new variables retain most of the information in the original variables, in the sense of accounting for a large part of their total variance.

In detail, the first principal component variable, y_1, is defined as that linear function of the original variables which accounts for the maximum amount of the variance of the original data amongst all possible linear functions. The second principal component, y_2, is defined as that linear function of the original variables which has maximum variance, *subject to being uncorrelated with y_1*. The remaining principal components are defined in the same way, each being a linear combination of the original variables with maximal variance, subject to being uncorrelated with the preceeding components. The p principal components, $y_1, y_2, \ldots, y_p$ are thus defined by

$$y_1 = a_{11}x_1 + a_{12}x_2 + \ldots + a_{1p}x_p$$
$$y_2 = a_{21}x_1 + a_{22}x_2 + \ldots + a_{2p}x_p$$
$$\vdots \tag{8.3}$$
$$y_p = a_{p1}x_1 + a_{p2}x_2 + \ldots + a_{pp}x_p$$

with the coefficients, $a_{ij}, i = 1, \ldots, p, j = 1, \ldots, p$ being chosen so that the maximum variance and uncorrelated conditions described above are achieved.

How are the coefficients calculated? Firstly, without some restrictions, the question cannot be answered, simply because each coefficient could be multiplied by some constant and the variance of each y variable increased without limit. The usual constraint imposed to overcome this problem is to require that the sum-of-squares of the coefficients defining each component equals one; that is $\sum_{j=1}^{p} a_{ij}^2 = 1$ for all i. This requirement may be written more concisely as

$$\mathbf{a}_i'\mathbf{a}_i = 1, i = 1, \ldots, p \tag{8.4}$$

where $\mathbf{a}_i'$ is a vector containing the coefficients defining the ith principal component, that is $\mathbf{a}_i' = [a_{i1}, a_{i2}, \ldots, a_{ip}]$. Alternative normalization constraints will be mentioned later.

Determining the coefficients which define the principal components involves finding quantities known as the *eigenvalues* (or latent roots), and *eigenvectors* (or latent vectors), of the sample covariance matrix, $\mathbf{S}$. A full explanation of these terms is given in Everitt and Dunn (1991), but for each eigenvalue there is a corresponding eigenvector and both can be found from $\mathbf{S}$. The largest eigenvalue, λ_1 and its corresponding eigenvector, $\mathbf{a}_1$, give, respectively, the variance of and the coefficients defining the first principal component. Similarly the coefficients defining the second principal component are found from the eigenvector, $\mathbf{a}_2$, corresponding to the second largest eigenvalue, λ_2.

In this way a set of p principal components variables are obtained which are uncorrelated and account for decreasing portions of the variance of the original variables.

But how useful are artificial variables constructed in this way? To answer this question it is necessary to know the proportion of variance of the original variables accounted for by each component (see below). If, for example, 80% of the variance in a data set with ten variables was accounted for by just the first two principal components, then a highly parsimonious summary of the data would have been achieved which might prove extremely useful in both describing the data concisely and in subsequent analyses. Examples will be given later.

The eigenvalues, $\lambda_1, \lambda_2, \ldots, \lambda_p$, give the variances of the derived variables, $y_1, y_2, \ldots, y_p$. The total variance of the derived variables is equal to the total variance of the original variables so that

$$\sum_{i=1}^{p} \lambda_i = \sum_{i=1}^{p} s_{ii} \tag{8.5}$$

The sum of the elements in the main diagonal of a matrix is usually called its *trace*, so that (8.5) may be rewritten as

$$\sum_{i=1}^{p} \lambda_i = \text{trace}(\mathbf{S}) \tag{8.6}$$

Consequently the jth principal component accounts for a proportion

$$\frac{\lambda_j}{\text{trace}(\mathbf{S})} \tag{8.7}$$

of the total variance in the original data, and the first p^* components account for a proportion

$$\frac{\sum_{i=1}^{p^*} \lambda_i}{\text{trace}(\mathbf{S})} \tag{8.8}$$

In many sets of multivariate data the variables will be measured in widely different units. The data in Table 8.1 provide such an example. In these cases linear combinations of the raw variable values will make little sense, and it is more usual to calculate the principal components after the original variables have been standardized to have a common scale, usually to have unit variance. This is equivalent to deriving the coefficients defining the components from the eigenvectors of the correlation matrix, $\mathbf{R}$, rather than from the covariance matrix, $\mathbf{S}$. It is important to realise however, that the eigenvalues and eigenvectors of $\mathbf{R}$ will not necessarily be at all similar to those of $\mathbf{S}$, and that choosing to use the former rather than the latter involves a definite, but perhaps arbitrary decision to make the variables 'equally important'. In a correlation matrix the diagonal terms are all unity so that its trace is equal to p, the number of variables in the data set. Consequently the proportion of the total variance accounted for by the jth component is now simply λ_j/p.

One of the questions that needs to be considered when carrying out a principal components analysis is 'how many components give an adequate summary of the data?' A number of relatively informal methods have been suggested. The most common are:

(1) include just enough components to explain say, 80% of the total variance;
(2) exclude those principal components whose variances are less than the average, that is, less than one, if a correlation matrix has been used;
(3) plot the value of λ_i against i for $i = 1, \ldots p$, and look for an 'elbow,' indicating where 'large' variances cease and 'small' variances begin. This is usually known as a *scree* plot.

Rules for indicating the number of components which have more sound statistical foundations have been suggested but Jolliffe (1986) concludes that these have, at present, little advantage over simpler methods. Jolliffe (1972) does however suggest that when using rule (2) above with a correlation matrix, a cutoff of 0.7 might be more useful then the usual value of 1.0.

The scores for each individual on each component are found by simply applying the appropriate set of coefficients to the relevant set of variable values. It is conventional to standardize the original variables to have zero means so that the resulting component scores also have zero means. If the components are derived from the correlation matrix then component scores are found from the original variable values after these have been standardized to have unit variance. If the first $p^*(p^* < p)$ components are judged to provide a reasonable summary of the data, then scores for each of the individuals on these components may be used in later analyses in place of the original variables.

Principal components are often scaled so that the sum of squares of their coefficients equal not unity but the corresponding eigenvalue. If the components are extracted from the correlation matrix, the rescaled coefficients represent *correlations* between the variables and the components. This form of scaling is often very useful in the interpretation of the components.

8.3.1 Examples of principal components analysis

It will be helpful to begin with a very simple example involving only two variables, height and weight. A data set of the heights and weights of 100 individuals is shown in the scattergram given in Figure 8.2. For two variables with correlation $r > 0$, it can be shown that the two principal component variables are given by

$$y_1 = \frac{1}{\sqrt{2}}(x_1 + x_2) \tag{8.9}$$

$$y_2 = \frac{1}{\sqrt{2}}(x_1 - x_2) \tag{8.10}$$

with the corresponding variances being given by $\lambda_1 = 1 + r, \lambda_2 = 1 - r$. Figure 8.3 again shows the scattergram of the height, weight measurements after standardisation of each variable to zero mean and unit variance. In addition Figure 8.3 shows the two principal component axes. (Mathematically principal components analysis is nothing more than a rotatation of the coordinate axes of a data set). The first component can be interpreted as a measure of an individuals 'size', separating large and small individuals, the second as a

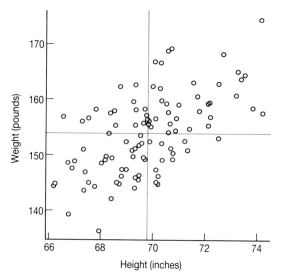

Figure 8.2 Scatterplot of height and weight measurements

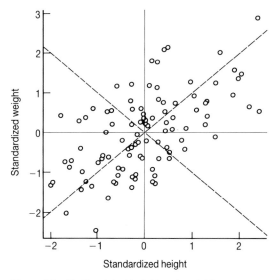

Figure 8.3 Scatterplot of height and weight measurements showing the two principal components of the correlation matrix

measure of 'shape', separating 'short/heavy' people from those who are tall and light.

As a further example of a principal components analysis, the method will be applied to the correlation matrix shown in Table 8.5, taken from Finn (1974). These correlations arose in a study concerned with dental calculus reduction. The six variables measured in this study were calculus accumulation

Table 8.5 Correlations of the calculus measurements for the six anterior mandibular teeth (reproduced with permission from Finn, 1974)

$$\mathbf{R} = \begin{array}{c} \\ 1 \\ 2 \\ 3 \\ 4 \\ 5 \\ 6 \end{array} \begin{array}{cccccc} 1 & 2 & 3 & 4 & 5 & 6 \\ \left(\begin{array}{cccccc} 1.00 & & & & & \\ 0.54 & 1.00 & & & & \\ 0.34 & 0.65 & 1.00 & & & \\ 0.37 & 0.65 & 0.84 & 1.00 & & \\ 0.36 & 0.59 & 0.67 & 0.80 & 1.00 & \\ 0.62 & 0.49 & 0.43 & 0.42 & 0.55 & 1.00 \end{array}\right) \end{array}$$

Variables are calculus measure on
1 Right canine,
2 Right lateral, incisor
3 Right central, incisor
4 Left central, incisor
5 Left lateral incisor
6 Left canine

Table 8.6 Principal components of the correlation matrix in Table 8.5

	PC1	*PC2*	*PC3*	*PC4*	*PC5*	*PC6*
1 Right canine	0.64	0.65	−0.23	−0.29	−0.13	0.04
2 Right lat.inc.	0.83	0.04	−0.41	0.38	−0.04	0.01
3 Right cen.inc.	0.84	−0.35	−0.09	−0.15	0.33	−0.15
4 Left cen.inc.	0.88	−0.37	0.00	−0.17	−0.05	0.25
5 Left lat.inc.	0.85	−0.22	0.32	0.05	−0.33	−0.14
6 Left canine	0.71	0.50	0.40	0.15	0.22	0.06
Variance	3.81	0.99	0.50	0.31	0.29	0.11

for six anterior teeth of the lower mandible. The coefficients defining the six principal component variables and their variances are shown in Table 8.6. Here the coefficients are scaled so that their sum-of-squares equals the corresponding eigenvalue. Consequently the coefficients represent correlations between components and observed variables.

The first component accounts for 63% of the variance of the standardized calculus measures and appears to represent a weighted average calculus accumulation, with the contribution to the component increasing as the teeth approach the front of the mouth. The second component, accounting for an additional 17% of the variance, is largely a comparison of incisors with the canines. The component probably reflects both differential usage in eating and brushing as well as proximity of the salivary glands. The third component accounts for a further 8% of the variance and reflects differences in calculus formation on the two sides of the mouth. It seems that there exists a tendency for individuals to have a greater calculus formation on one or other side of the mouth. This may reflect lateral favouritism in biting and/or brushing. The remaining three components account for only a total of 12% of the variance and might safely be ignored. Figure 8.4 shows a plot of the eigenvalues (vari-

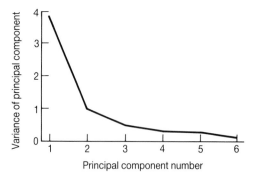

Figure 8.4   Scree plot of principal components of dental data

ances) which indicates that the first two or perhaps three components are of most importance.

A further fascinating example of principal components analysis is given in Jolliffe and Morgan (1992). The data in this case arose from an investigation of extradural haematoma, with twelve variables being observed on 172 patients. The corresponding correlation matrix and a description of the variables is given in Table 8.7.

The coefficients defining the first four components are shown in Table 8.8. The first two components account for 42% of the variance of the original variables. The first component appears to separate individuals with large time intervals (and consequent slow development of haematoma), no deep coma and good outcome, from those with small intervals (and consequent fast development of haematoma), deep coma and poor outcomes. The negative coefficient of age arises because age is correlated with outcome, younger individuals with more flexible skulls being expected to accommodate a swelling haematoma more easily without brain damage. The second principal component separates out individuals according to change in coma state between hospital arrival and prior to operation. High coma deterioration makes the score on this component large, as does a small interval and the presence of alcohol.

A principal components analysis can often provide an informative graphical display of a set of multivariate data. With the haematoma data for example, a plot of the first two principal component scores of each individual is shown in Figure 8.5. This plot reveals that high deterioration of the coma variables between the two occasions of measurement is far more common than otherwise. Additionally, the plot is, according to Jolliffe and Morgan, suggestive of two subgroups, corresponding roughly to good and poor outcomes. This type of principal component plot is often very useful for identifying outliers, or as here, indicating possible 'cluster' structure in the data which might be investigated further using some method of cluster analysis — see Chapter 9.

Table 8.7 Correlation matrix for the variables measured in the extradural haematoma study

	1	2	3	4	5	6	7	8	9	10	11	12
1	1.000											
2	0.004	1.000										
3	−0.020	0.034	1.000									
4	0.039	0.008	0.236	1.000								
5	0.153	−0.101	0.086	0.116	1.000							
6	−0.181	0.088	0.180	0.108	0.040	1.000						
7	0.179	−0.065	−0.141	−0.040	0.305	−0.028	1.000					
8	0.062	0.013	−0.598	−0.296	−0.037	−0.162	0.183	1.000				
9	0.175	−0.023	−0.197	−0.126	−0.236	−0.088	0.838	0.211	1.000			
10	0.070	−0.021	−0.561	−0.314	−0.040	−0.227	0.224	0.760	0.299	1.000		
11	0.077	0.061	0.165	0.114	−0.109	0.095	−0.047	−0.065	−0.090	−0.065	1.000	
12	0.390	0.002	−0.251	−0.131	0.099	−0.292	0.285	0.390	0.349	0.549	0.023	1.000

The variables measured were as follows:
1 Age
2 Sex
3 Interval between injury and treatment
4 Result of special test (e.g. whether or not skull was fractured)
5 Whether or not alcohol was present
6 Whether general anaesthesia was used in the operation
7 Best verbal response on admission to hospital
8 Best verbal response prior to operation
9 Best motor response on admission to hospital
10 Best motor response prior to operation
11 Distance, in miles, between referring hospital and the treating hospital
12 Outcome following operation.
The verbal and motor responses record coma state, and were measured on a scale from 1 (best: orientated and obeying commands), to 5 (worst: no response of either kind) and outcome was recorded on a scale from 1 (full recovery) to 6 (dead).

Table 8.8 First four principal components of the correlation matrix in Table 8.7

Variable	PC1	PC2	PC3	PC4
1	−2	−3	−6	1
2	0	1	−2	−6
3	4	−3	−2	0
4	2	−3	−2	0
5	−1	−5	1	2
6	2	−1	3	−5
7	−3	−5	2	−2
8	−4	3	0	−1
9	−3	−4	2	−2
10	−5	2	0	−1
11	1	0	−5	−5
12	−4	−1	−4	0

(Coefficients rounded to one decimal place and multiplied by 10)

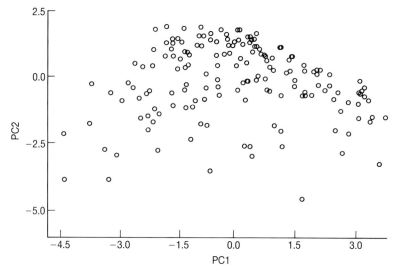

Figure 8.5   Plot of first two principal component scores from haematoma study

8.4 Factor analysis

Like principal components analysis, factor analysis attempts to reduce the dimensionality of a multivariate data set and often the results from two approaches are rather similar. The idea behind factor analysis is, however, quite different from principal component analysis. Factor analysis postulates that underlying the observed variables $x_1, x_2, \ldots, x_p$, there are m unobservable variables or *common factors*, $f_1, f_2, \ldots, f_m$. The observed variables are assumed to be linear combinations of the factors plus, for each variable, an error term or *specific factor*. Explicitly the assumed model can be written

$$x_j = \sum_{k=1}^{m} \lambda_{jk} f_k + e_j \qquad (8.11)$$

The common factors are assumed to be in standardized form with mean zero and unit variance. Often they are also assumed to be uncorrelated. The coefficient λ_{jk} is known as the *loading* of the jth variable on the kth common factor, and if $\psi_j = \mathrm{var}(e_j)$, then $1 - \psi_j$ is the *communality* of the jth variable, that is the proportion of the variation in x_j which is common to other observed variables, through their relationship to the common factors.

Full details of the factor analysis model are given in Everitt and Dunn (1991). Here it will suffice to note that to implement the method for a given value of m requires the factor loadings and communalities to be found, such that the correlations between the observed variables as predicted by the model are 'close' to the observed correlations. One problem with the factor analysis model which often gives rise to confusion, is that there is no unique solution for the loadings and communalities. It is this lack of uniqueness which gives rise to the process known as *rotation*, whereby the initial loadings extracted are 'rotated to simple structure' to make them as easy as possible to interpret. In practice this means making as many of the loadings as possible close to zero or ± 1.

Essentially then any factor analysis consists of two steps, finding an initial solution and then rotating that solution. Several methods of rotation are possible, one of the most commonly used being the *varimax* procedure — see Jolliffe and Morgan, 1992, for details. (It should be noted here that rotation is often also applied to principal component solutions. Although this may simplify the interpretation it must be realised that the rotated components no longer account for maximal proportions of the observed variance.)

To illustrate the use of factor analysis, a study reported by Whittick (1989) will be described. Attitudes to caregiving were examined in three groups of carers, namely mothers caring for a mentally handicapped child, mothers caring for a mentally handicapped adult and daughters caring for a parent with dementia. An attitude questionnaire was developed and administered by post to the three groups. The correlations between the 26 items on the questionnaire, derived from the returned questionnaires of 145 carers, were subjected to a factor analysis with varimax rotation. Table 8.9 presents the patterns of factor loadings on the first three factors. The three factors were interpreted as follows:

Factor 1: Negative aspects of caregiving with an emphasis on role conflict, family disruption and resentment about the caring role. This factor was labelled as 'conflict'.

Factor 2: Positive aspects of caregiving the emphasis on love for the dependent and satisfaction gained from the caregiving role. This factor was referred to as 'love'.

Factor 3: Willingness to accept institutional care with an emphasis on the advantages of institutional care. This factor was labelled 'institution'.

To represent these factors, three scales were created using items with a loading > 0.40, and such that a low score indicated an absence of the particular attitude and a high score indicated that the attitude was strongly held. Mean scores by care group for each attitude subscale were calculated and are shown in Table 8.10. A one-way analysis of variance showed that there were significant differences between care groups on all three subscales. (The relevant F values are shown in Table 8.10.) Daughters showed a higher mean score on subscales 'conflict' and 'institution' and a lower mean score on the 'love' subscale. Here the factor analysis has provided a very useful summary of a data set with a large number of variables.

Factor analysis as described above should more accurately be called *exploratory factor analysis*. The word 'exploratory' in this context implies that the investigator goes into the analysis with no preconceived ideas of what the factor structure should be, except the hope that it will be relatively simple and open to obvious interpretation. In some situations, however, the researcher would like to assess whether a set of variables conform to a factor analysis model with some particular structure, perhaps arising from theoretical considerations. In such cases the techniques of *confirmatory factor analysis* may be needed. Such models are often well described by a *path diagram* indicating

Table 8.9   Loadings on the first three factors for attitudes amongst carers

Item	F1	F2	F3
01 State should do more	0.16	0.19	−0.06
02 Relative to depend on me	−0.05	0.33	−0.14
03 Institution — good care and affection	0.20	−0.10	0.67
04 Others admire my care	−0.28	−0.03	−0.06
05 Euthanasia	−0.03	−0.07	0.08
06 Institution — good nursing care	0.21	−0.13	0.74
07 Care because of love	−0.06	0.50	−0.22
08 Abortion	0.02	−0.02	0.08
09 Others resent care	0.60	−0.05	0.14
10 Relative in institution	0.37	−0.26	0.65
11 Closer to relative	0.23	0.44	−0.16
12 Caring will be too much	0.61	−0.11	0.35
13 No-one else will care	0.49	−0.08	0.26
14 Death a release	0.26	−0.07	0.08
15 Others are neglected	0.50	−0.09	0.02
16 At a loss without relative	−0.20	0.68	−0.21
17 Provide more care	0.18	0.15	0.10
18 Family closer	−0.50	0.34	−0.12
19 Care single-handed	0.59	0.00	0.16
20 Feel closest to relative	0.06	0.56	−0.09
21 Consider institutional care	0.54	−0.23	0.48
22 Satisfaction from caring	−0.33	0.69	−0.11
23 Family's duty to care	−0.00	0.20	−0.08
24 Guilty if didn't care	−0.16	0.30	−0.02
25 Rather care than anything	−0.28	0.51	−0.07
26 Marriage problems	0.49	0.21	0.11

Table 8.10   Caregiving attitudes: subscale scores for each care group

Subscale	Mother/ child	Mother/ adult	Daughter/ parent	F
Conflict				
Mean	19.6	21.3	27.8	
SD	6.3	5.8	4.5	19.5
Love				
Mean	24.3	25.0	19.4	
SD	3.9	3.8	4.3	21.3
Institution				
Mean	7.5	8.3	12.9	
SD	3.5	2.9	2.7	34.5

the postulated connections between the observed variables and the factors. An example of a path diagram taken from Huba *et al.* (1981), is shown in Figure 8.6. Here the correlations between frequency of use of 13 substances by college students are postulated to arise from the relationships of the 13 observed or *manifest* variables to three underlying factors representing *alcohol use*, *cannabis use* and *hard drug use*. Full details of confirmatory factor analysis

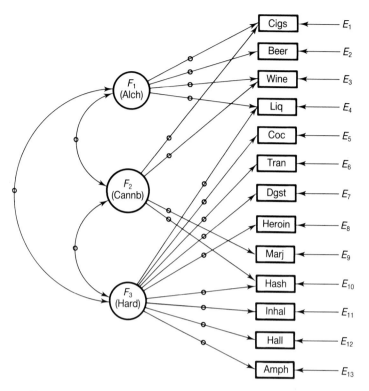

o = Free parameter to be estimated. Note paths between factors:
model allows observed variables which are not indicators of factors
to be correlated.

Figure 8.6 Path diagram for confirmatory factor analysis model for drug taking in college students

models, including an analysis of the Huba *et al.* data, are given in Dunn *et al.* (1993).

8.5 Correspondence analysis

A technique which is, in many ways closely similar to principal components analysis, but applicable to tables of counts is *correspondence analysis*, a method for deriving a set of coordinate values representing the row and columns of a contingency table and allowing the table to be displayed graphically. The correspondence analysis coordinates are analogous to those derived from a principal components analysis, except that they involve a partition of a chi-square statistic rather than total variance. In this section only a brief account of the method is given. A full account is available in Greenacre (1984).

Beginning with a two-dimensional contingency table of counts, such as that give in Table 8.11, the coordinates representing the row and column categories are derived from a matrix, E, with elements which are the residuals from fitting

Table 8.11   Hair colour and eye colour data

Eye colour	Fair	Red	Hair colour Medium	Dark	Black
Light	688	116	584	188	4
Blue	326	38	241	110	3
Medium	343	84	909	412	26
Dark	98	48	403	681	81

the independence model to the table, that is

$$e_{ij} = \frac{n_{ij} - E_{ij}}{\sqrt{E_{ij}}} \qquad (8.12)$$

where n_{ij} is the count in the ith row and jth column of the table and E_{ij} is the count expected if the row and column categories are independent. This expected value is given by

$$E_{ij} = \frac{n_{i.}n_{.j}}{n} \qquad (8.13)$$

where $n_{i.}$ and $n_{.j}$ are row and column marginal totals and n is the total number of observations

A procedure known as the *singular value decomposition* of E (see Everitt and Dunn, 1991), leads to two sets of coordinates, one set representing the rows of the table and the other the columns. Generally the first, or more often, the first two, coordinates for each row category and for each column category are used to display the table graphically. The adequacy or otherwise of such a display, is indicated by the proportion of the chi-square statistic for the table that it accounts for.

For a two-dimensional representation, the row category coordinates may be represented as $u_{ik}, i = 1,2,...,r, k = 1,2$ and the column categories as $v_{jk}, j = 1,2,...,c, k = 1,2$. It can be shown that a large positive residual corresponds to row and column coordinates which are large and of the same sign, a large negative residual to row and column coordinates which are large and of opposite signs, and a small residual to small coordinate values or to coordinates whose signs are not consistent for $k = 1$ and 2. A number of examples will help to clarify how the method is used.

Consider first the eye colour/hair colour data in Table 8.11. The overall chi-square statistic in this case is 1240. Clearly the two variables are not independent. The two-dimensional plot resulting from correspondence analysis is shown in Figure 8.7. These two coordinates account for 99% of the chi-square and so give an excellent representation of the data. The interpretation of the plot is very clear. Points representing dark eyes and dark hair are close to each other and some way from the origin, indicating a large positive residual in the corresponding cell of the table. Dark eyes and fair hair are represented by points on opposite sides of the origin and so the corresponding cell in the table has a large negative residual.

As a further example of the application of correspondence analysis consider the data in Table 8.12 on headache type by age taken from Greenacre (1992).

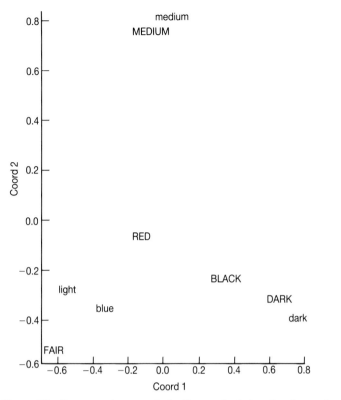

Figure 8.7 Correspondence analysis diagram for hair colour/eye colour data

The two-dimensional correspondence analysis solution is shown in Figure 8.8. The age groups trace a smooth 'trajectory' through this display, starting at the left, then moving down towards the right before bending upwards and back to the left. The three outlying headache category points act as references for interpreting the positions of the age groups, with the left hand side being identified with the category 'no diagnosis', the bottom right with 'migraine' and the top with 'tension headache'. Thus the youngest age group is the furthest towards the 'no diagnosis' pole of the display. The three middle age groups all tend in the direction of the 'migraine role' but amongst them there is a movement upwards the 'tension headache' pole as age increases. Finally the 50+ age group is closest to the 'tension headache' pole but has also moved back towards 'no diagnosis'.

Further interesting examples of the use of correspondence analysis in medical investigations are those reported in Leclerc *et al.* (1988) and Crichton and Hinde (1989).

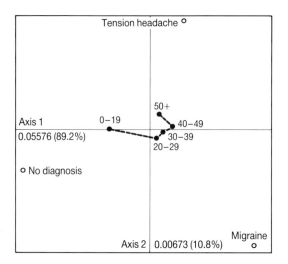

Figure 8.8   Correspondence analysis diagram for headache data

Table 8.12   Frequencies of headache types in 681 headache sufferers

Age group	None	Diagnosis Tension headache	Migraine	Total
0-19	77	52	20	149
20-29	66	82	68	216
30-39	31	49	37	117
40-49	20	44	31	95
50-59	27	52	25	104
Total	221	279	181	681

8.6 Summary

In this chapter, three methods useful for deriving summary variables for sets of multivariate data have been described. The first, and most widely used in medical research, is principal components analysis, a technique for transforming a set of variables into a new set of uncorrelated variables which account for maximal amounts of the variance of the original variables. Factor analysis, which often gives similar solutions to principal components analysis, also seeks a lower dimensional representation of the data, but postulates a formal model involving a small number of common factors, assumed to be responsible for generating the correlations between the observed variables. Factor analysis is widely used in the behavioural sciences, but less so in medicine, perhaps because the assumed model is often not considered realistic. Correspondence analysis leads to a graphical display of two-way tables of counts, with the coordinates derived in a similar fashion to the methods used in principal components analysis. This method is becoming more popular in medical investigations particularly when used to supplement other more formal methods of analysing categorical data (see, for example, Van der Heijden *et al.*, 1989).

9

Cluster Analysis

9.1 Introduction

Classification has played an important role in the development of many areas of science, most notably in biology, zoology and medicine. In the latter the classification of diseases has been fundamental for the progress which has occurred in the medical field during the post hundred years or so. Without it medicine would still be in the dark ages.

For a classification of diseases to be of any use it must first describe well patterns of similarities and differences among patients. A useful classificatory label will refer to a group of patients who have a rather similar pattern of symptoms when compared to each other, and a different pattern from patients with other labels. Description alone, however, is not a sufficient aim for medical classification, since it ignores such important areas as aetiology and treatment. A classification which grouped together patients suffering from yellow fever, meningitis and pneumonia, for example, would meet the descriptive requirement but would clearly not be a very useful classification, since aetiology and treatment have played no part in its construction. The most useful classifications for medical research will, in addition to providing convenient, parsimonious descriptions of patients with a variety of disorders, need to provide a basis for research into the causes of the disorder and have some relevance for treatment, in the sense that the classificatory labels are predictive of outcome. Many clinicians might regard the latter as the *most* important requirement of a classification scheme in medicine.

Statistical techniques for classification are essentially of two types. The first, known as *clustering techniques*, are used to construct a (hopefully) sensible and informative classification of an initial unclassified set of data, using the variable values observed on each individual. Paykel and Rassaby (1978), for example, studied 236 suicide attempters presenting at the main emergency service of one city in the United States. Each patient was described by 14 variables including age, number of previous suicide attempts, severity of depression, etc. A number of clustering methods were applied to the data and a final classification with three groups was produced which appeared potentially valuable as a basis for future studies into the causes and treatment of attempted suicide.

The second set of statistical techniques concerned with classification are known as *discriminant* or *assignment* methods. Here the classification scheme is known *a priori* and the problem is now to devise rules for assigning as yet unclassified individuals to one or other of the known classes. With a disease which can only be accurately diagnosed via a post-mortem examination, for example, it would obviously be desirable to have a method for allocating patients to either the disease or no-disease class, which minimizes the chance of misclassification and allows the appropriate therapeutic action to be taken whilst the patient is still alive. Such a rule might be derived from observations taken, prior to death, on patients now dead and thus eventually diagnosed without error. Details of how such allocation rules can be derived will be described in the next chapter. In the remainder of this chapter, attention is concentrated on clustering techniques and their application.

9.2 Distance and similarity measures

To begin the discussion, consider a set of patients suffering from liver failure each of whom has had measurements taken of the activity of *lactate dehydrogenase isoezyme five* (LDH5), and *lactate dehydrogenase isoenzyme three* (LDH3). The data may be plotted as a scattergram to gain insight into its structure etc. Two hypothetical scattergrams are shown in Figures 9.1 and 9.2. In the first the patients appear to belong to a single group, suggesting perhaps that they are all suffering from the same disease. In contrast, Figure 9.2, indicates that the patients fall into two distinct groups, indicating that they are suffering from two different complaints, here possibly two types of hepatitis, acute infectious hepatitis and hepatitis secondary infectious mononucleosis.

In this case the data have been 'clustered' by a simple visual examination of the scattergram. Identifying groups in this way involves an assessment of the relative *distances* between the points in the diagram; those that lie close to one another are placed in the same group. For data sets involving only two measurements on each individual this approach provides a very efficient clustering procedure, since the human eye/brain system is such an excellent pattern recognition device. With more than two measurements the problem is not so straightforward and more complex clustering techniques are generally needed. Many have been suggested, most of which operate on a matrix of inter-individual distances or similarities, where the latter quantities may be defined in a variety of ways.

9.2.1 Distance measures

The most familiar distance measure is, of course, Eucidean, since locally at least, we live in a Euclidean universe. When the distance between points A and B is referred to in everyday conversation it is generally Euclidean distance that is meant. To introduce the measure, consider Figure 9.3 The Euclidean distance between points i and j shown on the diagram, is, from Pythagoras'

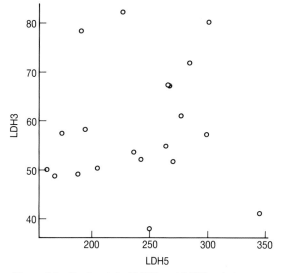

Figure 9.1 Scatterplot of LDH5 and LDH3 values

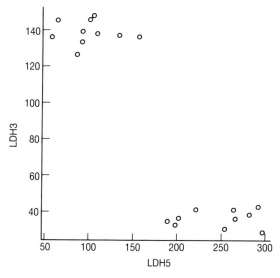

Figure 9.2 Scatterplot of LDH5 and LDH3 values

theorem, calculated as

$$d_{ij} = [(2.5 - 1.5)^2 + (2.5 - 1.5)^2]^{\frac{1}{2}} = 1.41 \tag{9.1}$$

When there are p variable values for each individual, Euclidean distance is defined as

$$d_{ij} = [(x_{i1} - x_{j1})^2 + (x_{i2} - x_{j2})^2 + \dots + (x_{ip} - x_{jp})^2]^{\frac{1}{2}} \tag{9.2}$$

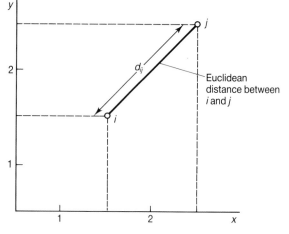

Figure 9.3 Euclidean distance in two dimensions

$$d_{ij} = \left[\sum_{k=1}^{p} (x_{ik} - x_{jk})^2 \right]^{\frac{1}{2}} \tag{9.3}$$

The Euclidean distances between each pair of individuals in a data set can be arranged in a matrix, **D**, which is *symmetric* (since $d_{ij} = d_{ji}$) with elements on the main diagnonal having value zero ($d_{ii} = 0$). It is such a matrix which is the starting point of many clustering procedures.

The calculation of a Euclidean distance matrix will be illustrated using the data on a small number of acidosis patients shown in Table 9.1. The Euclidean distance between patients 1 and 2 is given by

$$d_{12} = [(39.8 - 53.7)^2 + (38.0 - 37.2)^2 + (22.2 - 18.7)^2 + (23.2 - 18.5)^2]^{\frac{1}{2}} = 15.10 \tag{9.4}$$

The distances between the other pairs of individuals can be similarly calculated leading to the complete distance matrix, **D**

$$
\mathbf{D} = \begin{array}{c} 1 \\ 2 \\ 3 \\ 4 \\ 5 \\ 6 \end{array}
\begin{pmatrix}
\begin{array}{cccccc}
1 & 2 & 3 & 4 & 5 & 6 \\
0.00 & 15.01 & 7.85 & 2.14 & 5.61 & 8.20 \\
15.01 & 0.00 & 9.31 & 13.24 & 12.44 & 8.62 \\
7.85 & 9.31 & 0.00 & 6.10 & 3.44 & 2.24 \\
2.14 & 13.24 & 6.10 & 0.00 & 4.27 & 6.70 \\
5.61 & 12.44 & 3.44 & 4.27 & 0.00 & 4.58 \\
8.20 & 8.62 & 2.24 & 6.70 & 4.58 & 0.00
\end{array}
\end{pmatrix}
$$

Calculation of Euclidean distances from the raw data in this way may not always be sensible, because the variables may be on very different scales. This is certainly the case for the acidosis data, where the values of the Euclidean distances are largely dominated by the values on the first variable. In such cases a more acceptable, but still not a completely satisfactory alternative, is to standardize each variable to have unit variance before calculating the distances. If such a procedure is adopted for the acidosis data, the revised

Table 9.1 Data on acidosis patients

Patient	Variable 1	2	3	4
1	39.8	38.0	22.2	23.2
2	53.7	37.2	18.7	18.5
3	47.3	39.8	23.3	22.1
4	41.7	37.6	22.8	22.3
5	44.7	38.5	24.8	24.4
6	47.9	39.8	22.0	23.3

Variable
1. PH in cerebrospinal fluid (nanomol/litre)
2. PH in blood (nanomol/litre)
3. HCO_3 in cerebrospinal fluid (millimoles/litre)
4. HCO_3 in blood (millimoles/litre)

distance matrix, $\mathbf{D}_s$, becomes

$$\mathbf{D}_s = \begin{array}{c} \\ 1 \\ 2 \\ 3 \\ 4 \\ 5 \\ 6 \end{array} \begin{array}{cccccc} 1 & 2 & 3 & 4 & 5 & 6 \\ \left(\begin{array}{cccccc} 0.00 & & & & & \\ 4.06 & 0.00 & & & & \\ 2.40 & 4.04 & 0.00 & & & \\ 0.73 & 3.66 & 2.34 & 0.00 & & \\ 1.75 & 4.65 & 1.78 & 1.74 & 0.00 & \\ 2.30 & 3.78 & 1.05 & 2.43 & 1.97 & 0.00 \end{array}\right) \end{array}$$

Comparing the two matrices $\mathbf{D}$ and $\mathbf{D}_s$ shows that the ordering of the distances has altered, a change which has obvious implications in a clustering context. The question of scaling in cluster analysis (as in multivariate analysis in general, see Chapter 8), raises some difficult problems which are discussed in detail in Everitt (1993), who also describes other possible distance measures for use in clustering.

9.2.2 Similarity measures

In some instances measures of *similarity* between pairs of individuals rather than distances are calculated. These measures are such that large values indicate two individuals who are alike with respect to their variable values. Similarity measures are often scaled to be between zero and one. Many such measures are available but the most widely used are those appropriate for binary variables. Such data, for two individuals, may be arranged in the form of a 2×2 table as follows.

		Individual i		Total
		1	0	
Individual j	1	a	b	$a+b$
	0	c	d	$c+d$
	Total	$a+c$	$b+d$	$a+b+c+d=p$

Table 9.2 Similarity coefficients for binary data

(i)	$\frac{a+d}{p}$	(ii)	$\frac{a}{a+b+c}$
(iii)	$\frac{2a}{2a+b+c}$	(iv)	$\frac{2(a+d)}{2(a+d)+b+c}$
(v)	$\frac{a}{a+2(b+c)}$	(vi)	$\frac{a}{p}$

Here a, b, c and d represent counts of numbers of matches and mismatches on the binary variables. (The 2×2 table as used in clustering applications is primarily a convenient way of arranging the data and should not be confused with the usual 2×2 contingency table.) Many similarity coefficients have been proposed that combine the quantities a, b, c and d. A number of these are listed in Table 9.2. More extensive lists are given in Sneath and Sokal (1973), Anderberg (1973) and Gower (1985).

The two coefficients most commonly used in practice are the simple matching coefficient (coefficient (i) in Table 9.2) and Jaccard's coefficient (coefficient (ii) in Table 9.2). The first is simply the ratio of the total number of variables on which the two individuals match, to the total number of variables. The second is the corresponding ratio when the number of '0,0' matches is ignored. The problem of whether or not to include the latter is of concern only when the variables are genuinely of the 'present' 'absent' variety. In such cases it might not be reasonable to consider two individuals as similar simply because they both *lack* a number of characteristics. (One of the examples described later illustrates this point.)

9.3 Hierarchical clustering techniques

Given a similarity or distance matrix there are a vast number of clustering techniques which could be applied to derive a classification of the individuals. Here a particular class of methods, *hierarchical clustering techniques*, will be of concern. All members of this class have in common that they proceed by a series of steps in which individuals, and later groups of individuals formed earlier in the procedure, are successively clustered together into larger and larger groups. The initial stage is that where each individual is considered as a single member 'group', and the final stage consists of a single cluster containing all the individuals. Investigators have then to decide which of the classifications best fits their data. Essentially this involves the difficult and largely unresolved problem of choosing the correct number of clusters. The problem is discussed in detail in Everitt (1979, 1993) and Milligan and Cooper (1985). At each particular stage of the hierarchical clustering process the two individuals, or two groups of individuals which are closest (or most similar) are fused into a single cluster. It is the different criteria which are used to determine inter-group distances that give rise to the variety of hierarchical clustering techniques available. Two will now be described in a little more detail — *single linkage* and *Ward's method*.

9.3.1 Single linkage clustering

This method arises from defining distance between group as the distance between their closest members. To illustrate the use of single linkage clustering it will be applied to the distance matrix $\mathbf{D}_s$ arising from the acidosis data in Table 9.1 after standardization. The first step in producing a single linkage hiearchical classification of the six individuals is to fuse the two individuals who are closest. This leads to individuals one and four being grouped together giving at this stage, five groups with membership as follows:

$$[1, 4] \quad [2] \quad [3] \quad [5] \quad [6]$$

A new distance matrix may now be formed giving distances between the two member group and the other individuals in addition to the remaining inter-individual distances. The former are calculated from

$$d_{(14)2} = \min[d_{12}, d_{42}] = d_{42} = 3.66 \tag{9.5}$$

$$d_{(14)3} = \min[d_{13}, d_{43}] = d_{43} = 2.34 \tag{9.6}$$

etc. The new distance matrix becomes

$$
\mathbf{D}_s^{(1)} =
\begin{array}{c}
(14) \\
2 \\
3 \\
5 \\
6
\end{array}
\begin{pmatrix}
(14) & 2 & 3 & 5 & 6 \\
0.00 & & & & \\
3.66 & 0.00 & & & \\
2.40 & 4.04 & 0.00 & & \\
1.74 & 4.65 & 1.78 & 0.00 & \\
2.30 & 3.78 & 1.05 & 1.97 & 0.00
\end{pmatrix}
$$

The smallest entry in this matrix is for individuals three and six, so these now become a further group of two individuals and a new distance matrix is again formed. In it the distance between the two groups now in existence is found from

$$d_{(14)(36)} = \min[d_{13}, d_{16}, d_{43}, d_{46}] = d_{43} = 2.34 \tag{9.7}$$

The procedure is repeated until all the individuals are joined into a single group. The whole process can be summarized in the form of diagram known as a *dendrogram*, which shows the fusions which have occurred at each step. The dendrogram for single linkage applied to the acidosis data is shown in Figure 9.4.

9.3.2 Ward's hierarchical clustering method

Ward (1963) proposed a clustering procedure in which at each step in the hierarchical clustering, fusion of every possible pair of clusters is considered and the two clusters whose union results in the minimum increase in *information loss* are combined. The latter is defined by Ward in terms of an error sum-of-squares criterion, ESS.

The rationale behind Ward's proposal can be illustrated most simply by considering a set of univariate data. Suppose, for example, 10 individuals have scores [2, 6, 2, 5, 6, 2, 2, 0, 0, 0] on some particular variable. The loss of information that would result from treating the ten individuals as belonging

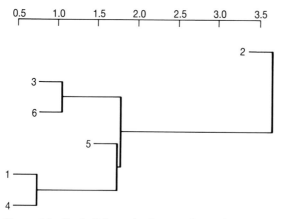

Figure 9.4   Single linkage dendrogram for acidosis data

to say, a single group, with mean 2.5 is measured by ESS as

$$ESS = \sum_{i=1}^{n}(x_i - \bar{x})^2 \qquad (9.8)$$

In this example then the value would be

$$ESS_{\text{one group}} = (2 - 2.5)^2 + (6 - 2.5)^2 + \ldots + (0 - 2.5)^2 = 50.5 \qquad (9.9)$$

Similarly if the 10 individuals are classified according to their scores into the following four groups

$$[0, 0, 0], [2, 2, 2, 2], [5], [6, 6]$$

the ESS can be evaluated as the sum of four separate error sum-of-squares

$$ESS_{\text{four groups}} = ESS_{\text{group one}} + ESS_{\text{group two}} + ESS_{\text{group three}} + ESS_{\text{group four}} = 0.0 \qquad (9.10)$$

Everitt (1993) discusses the properties and problems of hierarchical clustering methods in detail. In empirical investigations of the methods, see for example, Edelbrook (1979) and Milligan (1980), Ward's method has been found to be the most successful general-purpose hierarchical cluster method. Two medical applications of the method are now described.

9.3.3 The classification of lower back pain

Coste *et al.* (1991) describe an investigation of the clinical and psychological diversity of non-specific low-back pain. One aspect of the study involved the use of Ward's clustering method to produce a classification of 330 subjects complaining of localized low back pain to hospital rheumatologists. The variables recorded for each subject included information on their medical and surgical history, past and present back symptoms, intensity and duration of pain, type of onset, aggravating and relieving factors and activities. Cluster analysis was applied not to the raw data, but to standardized scores from a principal components analysis. On the basis of clinical judgement, the

Table 9.3 Exploratory classification of lower back pain (LBP): distribution of selected clinical features across the four classes

Cluster	1	2	3	4	*All*
No. of observations	46	194	70	19	329*
Mean age (yr)	56	46	51	54	49
Sex (% men)	40	53	33	10	45
Compensation status (%)	17	9	13	5	11
Median duration of LBP (weeks)	53	31	68	36	43
Previous separate attacks (> 0)(%)	100	33	97	58	42
Sudden onset (%)	21	30	23	15	26
In morning, back worse (%)	82	62	70	38	65
Permanent pain in night (%)	13	5	6	10	7
Diffuse spinal pain (%)	8	14	10	21	13
Pain increased by impulsion (%)	54	39	35	35	40
Pain worse on moving back (%)	90	70	75	47	72
Pain worse on standing (%)	65	52	60	42	54
pain worse with changing climate (%)	44	24	35	12	30
Pain worse by psychologic factors (%)	16	26	20	85	27
Dysethesias in the back (%)	4	10	6	40	10
Structural accentuated lordosis (%)	21	5	15	10	10
Spondylolisthesis hole (%)	17	3	6	5	7
Limited passive movements (%)	63	50	73	31	55
Catch (%)	26	15	13	5	15
Paravertebral muscular contracture (%)	21	14	15	0	15
Straight leg raising $< 75°$ (%)	40	31	35	0	30
DSM-III diagnosis[†] (%)	26	44	40	58	41

* Cluster analysis on 329 subjects. One subject was excluded because of unknown number of previous separate attacks of LBP.
[†] This variable did not participate in any way in the clustering process.

four-class partition produced by Ward's technique was deemed most useful. The profiles of the four classes on the original variables are shown in Table 9.3. The first cluster, consisting of 46 patients, was characterized by frequent mechanical features (pain increased by movements, impulsion, standing, lifting and relieved by lying; worst pain on the morning). Conversely, non-organic signs (diffuse spinal pain, dysesthesias, increased pain by psychological factors) were very uncommon. The fourth cluster described in Table 9.3 consisted of 19 patients who had the opposite characteristics to group one, namely, uncommon mechanical factors and physical findings, frequent non-organic signs. The second and third clusters appeared to be intermediate between the first and fourth. The clusters were further examined in terms of the prevalence of psychiatric disorders, and other cluster analyses performed on patients with and without psychiatric disorders. Clusters were eventually interpreted through the relationships or interactions between psychological disturbances and the clinical feature of low-back pain.

9.3.4 Developing a classification for facial pain

Wastell and Gray (1987) describe the use of clustering for the development of a classification of pain distribution in patients with temporomandibular joint pain dysfunction syndrome (TMJPDS). This refers to a complex symptom group involving facial pain, limitation and deviation of mandibular movements, joint noises and muscle tenderness. Symptoms vary with the stage of the disease. Aetiology is equally complex and both physical and psychogenic factors have been implicated. Pain is the most commonly recorded symptom but its facial distribution does not conform to a single pattern.

Wastell and Gray's main aim was to use clustering to develop an objective typology for classifying facial pain in terms of its spatial distribution. Clinically the hope was that the derived classification would be useful in identifying different stages of the disease, which would be helpful in defining more directed treatment plans. Data were collected from 127 patients attending the temporomandibular joint clinic of a University hospital complaining of classic TMJPDS. Patients were asked to trace the boundary of their pain affected area with the tip of their index finger. The examiner recorded this outline on a diagram of the lateral profile of the face (see Figure 9.5) and this was adjusted until patient were satisfied that the outline matched their own pain area. The squares of the grid shown in Figure 9.5 falling within the perimeter of a pain area were scored one, those without were scored zero. In this way any patients pain distribution could be described by a string of binary variables. In practice all distributions lay within a central rectangle with horizontal extension J–T and vertical extension 11–28, giving $11 \times 18 = 198$ binary variables for analysis. The similarity matrix calculated from these data was Jaccard's coefficient (see Section 9.2), the rationale being that in this case it is sensible to disregard '0,0' matches,

The dendrogram resulting from applying Ward's method to the derived similarity matrix is shown in Figure 9.6 The structure of the dendrogram appears to indicate three major classes, with a further possible subdivision of each of these into two. A composite pain distribution matrix for each class was constructed by simple matrix addition of the pain matrices of its constituent members. The description of the pain classes given by the authors was as follows.

Pain Class A: The pain distribution of Class A was concentrated over the temporomandibular joint (see Figure 9.7). The two subclasses were much alike, save for a small vertical difference in their centroids.

Pain Class B: The pain distribution of Class A differed from Class B in involving the vertical portion of the mandible (the ramus). The two subclasses of B were quite different; Class B2 showed a distribution confined to the lower part of the ramus and Class B1 a much wider distribution covering all the ramus and the interior part of the temple (see Figure 9.7).

Pain Class C: The pain distribution of Class C differed from the other two classes in involving an anterior projection over the zygomatic arch. The two subclasses were again distinct. Class C1 showed a distribution confined to the temporomandibular joint and the zygomatic arch; Class C2 showed a much wider distribution spreading over the temple as well as covering the ramus (Figure 9.7).

Wastell and Gray went to much effort to validate their proposed classification

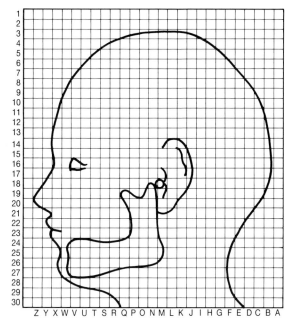

Figure 9.5 Lateral profile chart (for left side). The outline of the mandible is superimposed on the chart and the measurement grid is shown.

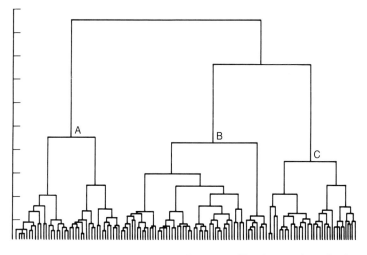

Figure 9.6 The dendrogram for Ward's method. The three major pain classes A, B and C are indicated

using a variety of methods, one of which was to relate the clusters found to clinical features. Many such features showed large differences between clusters. The final conclusion was that the cluster solution could be interpreted in terms of a chronological model of the development of TMJPDS.

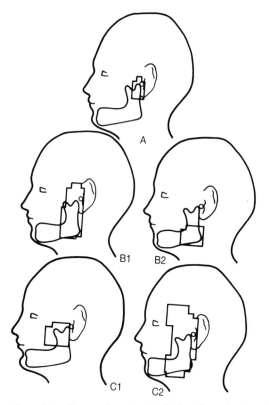

Figure 9.7 Composite pain distribution for pain class A and the two subclasses of B(B1 and B2) and the two subclasses of C (C1 and C2)

9.4 Clustering by fitting mixture distributions

The cluster analysis methods described in the previous section are unsatisfactory from a statistical viewpoint since they are not based on any well defined model of cluster structure. In addition they involve a number of decisions over scaling and choice of similarity or distance measure, all of which may affect the final cluster solution. A more statisfactory statistical approach to the clustering problem is provided by assuming that within each cluster the variation of the p variables is described by a probability density function of some form. The combined observations from several clusters will then have what is termed a *mixture* density. The problem now becomes one of identifying and describing the component densities using a sample drawn from the mixture.

In mathematical terms the approach may be formulated as follows. Assume that there are k clusters in the population and that within cluster i, the vector of observed variables arises from a probability density function.

$$g(\mathbf{x};\boldsymbol{\theta}_i) \tag{9.11}$$

where $\boldsymbol{\theta}_i$ is an m-dimensional vector of parameters. (If g was the univariate normal density for example, θ would contain the mean and standard deviation parameters that characterise the density.) If cluster i forms a proportion, p_i of the population, then the overall density function of $\mathbf{x}$ is given by

$$f(\mathbf{x}) = \sum_{i=1}^{k} p_i g(\mathbf{x}; \theta_i) \qquad (9.12)$$

where $0 < p_i < 1$, and $\sum_{i=1}^{k} p_i = 1$. The function $f(\mathbf{x})$ is known as a *finite mixture density*. The problem now is, given a sample of values, $\mathbf{x}_1, \mathbf{x}_2, \ldots, \mathbf{x}_n$ assumed to come from a population with density function $f(\mathbf{x})$, find estimates of the mixing proportions, $p_i, i = 1, \ldots, k$ and the parameter vectors, $\theta_i, i = 1, \ldots, k$. Given these estimates, individuals may be formed into clusters on the basis of the largest of the estimated posterior probabilities.

$$P(\text{cluster } s | \mathbf{x}_i) = \frac{\hat{p}_i g(\mathbf{x}_i; \hat{\theta}_s)}{\sum_{j=1}^{k} \hat{p}_j g(\mathbf{x}_i; \hat{\theta}_j)} \qquad (9.13)$$

for $s = 1, \ldots, k$.

Before considering how the parameters in (9.12) might be estimated, consideration needs to be given to useful specific forms for the component densities, $g(\mathbf{x}; \theta_i)$. This will depend on the type of variable being used. Two cases which are of most interest are

(1) when the variables are all continuous,
(2) when the variables are all categorical.

In the first case it is generally assumed that the component densities are multivariate normal so that the parameter vector, θ_i consists of the elements of the mean vector and the covariance matrix of the ith cluster. This case has been discussed in detail by Wolfe (1970), Day (1969), Everitt and Hand (1981) and McLachlan and Basford (1988).

When the variables are binary, one possibility which has been suggested is to assume that within clusters the variables are independent of one another leading to component densities of the form

$$g(\mathbf{x}; \theta_i) = \prod_{i=1}^{p} \theta_{ij}^{x_j} (1 - \theta_{ij})^{(1-x_j)} \qquad (9.14)$$

where now the elements of θ_i, that is $(\theta_{i1}, \theta_{i2}, \ldots, \theta_{ip})$, represent the probability of a particular variable taking the value one and $x_1, x_2, \ldots, x_p$ are the elements of $\mathbf{x}$. Such an approach to the clustering of binary data is often known as *latent class analysis* (see Lazarsfeld and Henry, 1968). The model is easily extended to categorical variables with more than two categories — see Goodman (1974) for details.

The parameters in these finite mixture models are generally estimated by maximum likelihood methods. Details are given in Everitt and Hand (1981), Chapters 2 and 5. Here a medical example of each type of mixture model will be described.

9.4.1 Fitting mixtures of multivariate normal densities to psychiatric data

During the last 20 years many attempts have been made to refine, replace and to validate intuitive clinical classifications of mental illness through the statistical analysis of symptom ratings. A number of these have involved the application of various methods of cluster analysis, and in Everitt *et al.* (1971), the fitting of multivariate normal densities was used as part of an investigation attempting to validate traditional psychiatric syndromes. Two sets of patients were used, one from the United Kingdom and the other from the United States of America. Both sets contained 250 patients. Each patient was described by 70 variables, a combination of mental state and history information. Before applying clustering each data set was subjected to a principal components analysis, and the first ten principal component scores of each patient calculated. It was these scores which were used as the basis for clustering the patients. The groups found in each data set were examined in terms of their psychiatric diagnostic labels. Four groups in each data set were relatively homogeneous in terms of these labels; the first was composed predominantly of patients with manic-depressive illness, the second patients with psychotic depressions, the third patients diagnosed as paranoid schizophrenic and the fourth, largely patients with chronic schizophrenic diagnosis. There were, however, a number of groups which contained patients with a variety of diagnostic labels; a surprising finding was the failure of patients diagnosed with neurotic depression to appear as a separate group, despite there being over 60 patients with this diagnosis in the two data sets.

9.4.2 The use of latent class analysis to form a classification of Scottish infants

A central issue in the allocation of hospital resources among regions or areas is the measurement of their differing need for medical services. One approach is to classify individuals into groups with similar medical characteristics and to use the prevalence of these groups as a basis for estimating the resources required by each area. Pickering and Forbes (1984) report the use of latent class analysis to form the initial classification of such an approach to the allocation of neonatal resources throughout Scotland. The data for analysis consisted of 11 categorical variables observed on 45 426 cases. The variables contained clinical and diagnostic information extracted from the Scottish Neonatal Discharge Record. Two, three and four class models were fitted using the usual approach to maximum likelihood estimation, the EM algorithm (see Goodman, 1974). The results of the analysis are shown in Table 9.4. Of the solutions shown, that with four classes was considered by the investigators as the most interesting and relevant. One class was associated with healthy infants, two others with moderately ill infants requiring various types of special neonatal care and the third representing severely ill, very low birthweight infants. The use of the classification is discussed in detail in the original paper.

Table 9.4 Classification of Scottish infants. Parameter estimates for one to four class models using 1980 data and complete cases only. (Reproduced with permission from Pickering and Forbes, 1984)

Vari-able	No of levels	Levels‡	1 class I	2 classes IIa	IIb	3 classes IIIa	IIIb	IIIc	4 classes IVa	IVb	IVc	IVd
1	4	2001–2500 g	0.05	0.01	0.48	0.00	0.18	0.79	0.00	0.20	0.78	0.03
		1501–2000 g	0.01	0.00	0.15	0.00	0.26	0.09	0.00	0.32	0.09	0.00
		⩽ 1500 g	0.01	0.00	0.08	0.00	0.21	0.01	0.00	0.25	0.01	0.00
2	2	< 10th centile	0.10	0.07	0.43	0.07	0.19	0.62	0.07	0.21	0.62	0.10
3	2	< 7	0.02	0.01	0.12	0.01	0.26	0.01	0.00	0.21	0.01	0.32
4	3	Intermediate*	0.09	0.08	0.19	0.08	0.26	0.13	0.07	0.25	0.13	0.31
		By intubation	0.03	0.02	0.17	0.02	0.33	0.04	0.01	0.29	0.00	0.52
5	2	Present	0.01	0.00	0.10	0.00	0.25	0.00	0.00	0.29	0.00	0.01
6	2	Present	0.01	0.00	0.06	0.00	0.17	0.00	0.00	0.20	0.00	0.00
7	2	Present	0.30	0.28	0.58	0.28	0.67	0.49	0.28	0.71	0.49	0.32
8	2	Present	0.00	0.00	0.03	0.00	0.07	0.00	0.00	0.07	0.00	0.01
9	2	Present	0.03	0.01	0.30	0.01	0.60	0.10	0.01	0.67	0.10	0.05
10	2	Present	0.00	0.00	0.05	0.00	0.13	0.00	0.00	0.15	0.00	0.00
11	3	4–10 days	0.80	0.84	0.34	0.83	0.09	0.53	0.83	0.04	0.50	0.84
		> 11 days	0.08	0.03	0.61	0.03	0.79	0.45	0.03	0.82	0.46	0.14
Frequency of class			1.00	0.92	0.08	0.92	0.03	0.05	0.89	0.03	0.05	0.04

Key:

1 Birthweight	4 Resuscitation	7 Jaundice†	10 Dead at discharge
2 Birthweight for gestation age	5 Assisted ventilation after 30 min	8 Convulsions	11 Age at discharge
3 Apgar at 5 min	6 Recurrent apnoea	9 In tube feeding	

* mask + intermittent positive pressure ventilation, Drugs only, Other

† > 86 μmol/litre bilirubin

‡ parameters for all levels of a variable sum to 1, the first level is omitted without loss of information

9.5 Summary

The literature on cluster analysis is vast and in this chapter only a flavour of the area has been given in an attempt to illustrate its potential. Many problems have been mentioned only in passing or have not been referred to at all. For more details readers are referred to Cormack (1971), Hartigan (1975) and Everitt (1979, 1993). In medicine clustering techniques have been most applied in psychiatry in an attempt to refine traditional psychiatric syndromes. Applications of the techniques in other areas of medicine are less common, although interesting examples may be found in Wong *et al.* (1983), Wastell (1985) and Spiegelhalter and Knill-Jones (1984).

10

Assignment Techniques

10.1 Introduction

Like Chapter 9, this one also deals with classification in medicine. Here, however, the interest is not in exploring a set of multivariate data for evidence of the existence of separate groups of individuals, but in deriving rules for allocating new patients to one of a set of *a priori* defined disease classes or diagnostic groups in some optimal way. Each such *assignment* or *discrimination* technique has as its basis, a series of variables collected from patients whose diseases have already been confirmed. These data serve to establish the characteristics of each disease group. A new patient is then diagnosed by determining in some way or other how typical their individual patterns of signs and symptoms is of each disease group in a turn. A variety of assignment procedures are available, no single method being optimal in all situations. Choice of method is governed by a number of considerations such as the number of measurements made on each patient, whether the variables describing each patient are measured on categorical or continuous scales, whether there are missing data etc. The most commonly used assignment techniques in a medical context are Fisher's *linear discriminant function* and *linear logistic discrimination* which is essentially equivalent to the logistic regression model described in Chapter 5. Both methods will now be described in more detail.

10.2 The linear discriminant function

The linear discriminant function was originally derived by Fisher (1936) as a technique for classifying an individual into one of two possible groups, on the basis of a set of observations or measurements, $x_1, x_2, \ldots, x_p$. Fisher's approach to the problem was to seek a linear transformation of the variables

$$z = a_1 x_1 + a_2 x_2 + \ldots + a_p x_p \tag{10.1}$$

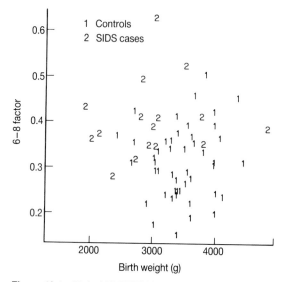

Figure 10.1   Plot of FACTOR68 values and BIRTHWEIGHT for SIDS data

such that the separation between the group means on the transformed scale, $\bar{z}_1$ and $\bar{z}_2$, would be maximized relative to the within-group variation on the z scale. The coefficients, $a_1, a_2, \ldots, a_p$ that achieve this requirement can be shown to be given by

$$\mathbf{a} = \mathbf{S}^{-1}(\bar{\mathbf{x}}_1 - \bar{\mathbf{x}}_2) \tag{10.2}$$

where $\mathbf{a}' = [a_1, a_2, \ldots, a_p]$, and $\mathbf{S}$ is the pooled within-groups covariance matrix of the two groups, calculated from the separate group covariance matrices, $\mathbf{S}_1$, and $\mathbf{S}_2$ as

$$\mathbf{S} = \frac{1}{n_1 + n_2}[n_1\mathbf{S}_1 + n_2\mathbf{S}_2] \tag{10.3}$$

where n_1 and n_2 are the sample sizes in each group. $\bar{\mathbf{x}}_1$ and $\bar{\mathbf{x}}_2$ are the mean vectors of the two groups.

To illustrate the use of Fisher's linear discriminant function, the data shown in Table 10.1 will be used. These data were collected by Spicer *et al.* (1987) in an investigation of sudden infant death syndrome (SIDS). The two groups here consist of 16 SIDS victims and 49 controls. The FACTOR68 variable arises from spectral analysis of 24 hour recordings of electrocardiograms and respiratory movements made on each child — see the original paper for more details. (The SIDS victims and the controls were matched for the age at which this recording was made). All the infants has a gestational age of 37 or more weeks and were regarded as full term.

To begin, only the FACTOR68 variable and BIRTHWEIGHT will be used. Table 10.2 shows the means of each of these variables for the cases and controls, and the pooled within-group covariance matrix. A scatterplot of the two variables with cases and controls identified is shown in Figure 10.1. The discriminant function coefficients calculated using (10.2) are 0.001 948

Table 10.1 SIDS data

Group	1	2	3	4
1	115.6	3060	0.291	39
1	108.2	3570	0.277	40
1	114.2	3950	0.390	41
1	118.8	3480	0.339	40
1	76.9	3370	0.248	39
1	132.6	3260	0.342	40
1	107.7	4420	0.310	42
1	118.2	3560	0.220	40
1	126.6	3290	0.233	38
1	138.0	3010	0.309	40
1	127.0	3180	0.355	40
1	127.7	3950	0.309	40
1	106.8	3400	0.250	40
1	142.1	2410	0.368	38
1	91.5	2890	0.223	42
1	151.1	4030	0.364	40
1	127.1	3770	0.335	42
1	134.3	2680	0.356	40
1	114.9	3370	0.374	41
1	118.1	3370	0.152	40
1	122.0	3270	0.356	40
1	167.0	3520	0.394	41
1	107.9	3340	0.250	41
1	134.6	3940	0.422	41
1	137.7	3350	0.409	40
1	112.8	3350	0.241	39
1	131.3	3000	0.312	40
1	132.7	3960	0.196	40
1	148.1	3490	0.266	40
1	118.9	2640	0.310	39
1	133.7	3630	0.351	40
1	141.0	2680	0.420	38
1	134.1	3580	0.366	40
1	135.5	3800	0.503	39
1	148.6	3350	0.272	40
1	147.9	3030	0.291	40
1	162.0	3940	0.308	42
1	146.8	4080	0.235	40
1	131.7	3520	0.287	40
1	149.0	3630	0.456	40
1	114.1	3290	0.284	40
1	129.2	3180	0.239	40
1	144.2	3580	0.191	40
1	148.1	3060	0.334	40
1	108.2	3000	0.321	37
1	131.1	4310	0.450	40
1	129.7	3975	0.244	40
1	142.0	3000	0.173	40
1	145.5	3940	0.304	41
2	139.7	3740	0.409	40
2	121.3	3005	0.626	38
2	131.4	4790	0.383	40
2	152.8	1890	0.432	38
2	125.6	2920	0.347	40
2	139.5	2810	0.493	39

Table 10.1 *continued*

Group	1	2	3	4
2	117.2	3490	0.521	38
2	131.5	3030	0.343	37
2	137.3	2000	0.359	41
2	140.9	3770	0.349	40
2	139.5	2350	0.279	40
2	128.4	2780	0.409	39
2	154.2	2980	0.388	40
2	140.7	2120	0.372	38
2	105.5	2700	0.314	39
2	121.7	3060	0.405	41

Group 1 = Controls, group 2 = cases.
1 = HEARTRATE
2 = BIRTHWEIGHT(g)
3 = FACTOR68
4 = GESAGE

Table 10.2 Means and pooled covariance matrix for
SIDS data FACTOR68 and BIRTHWEIGHT

Means

Variable	Controls	Cases
BIRTHWEIGHT	3437.86	2964.69
FACTOR68	0.31	0.40

Covariance matrix

	BIRTHWEIGHT	FACTOR68
BIRTHWEIGHT	278612.28	
FACTOR68	4.32	0.0062

and -16.0846, giving

$$z = 0.001\,948 \times \text{BIRTHWEIGHT} - 16.0846 \times \text{FACTOR68} \qquad (10.4)$$

To derive the classification rule the group means on the transformed variable are needed. These are obtained by simply applying the discriminant function coefficients to the group mean vectors, that is

$$\bar{z}_1 = 0.001\,948 \times 3437.857 - 16.0846 \times 0.310\,82 = 1.696 \qquad (10.5)$$
$$\bar{z}_2 = 0.001\,948 \times 2964.688 - 16.0846 \times 0.401\,81 = -0.6887 \qquad (10.6)$$

If an individual has a discriminant score which is closer to $\bar{z}_1$ than $\bar{z}_2$ then assignment is to the first group (the controls here); in the reverse situation assignment is to the second group (the SIDS). This classification rule can be formalized by defining a cut-off value z_c given by

$$z_c = \frac{\bar{z}_1 + \bar{z}_2}{2} \qquad (10.7)$$

Here $z_c = 0.5036$. Now (assuming as here that $\bar{z}_1 > \bar{z}_2$), the classification rule for an individual with discriminant score, z_i is

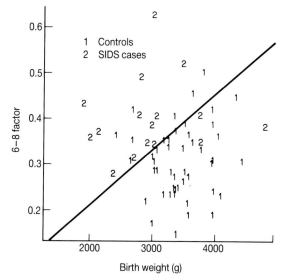

Figure 10.2 SIDS data showing derived Fisher's discriminant function

Assign subject to group one if $z_i - z_c > 0$
Assign subject to group two if $z_i - z_c \leqslant 0$

The discriminant function can be plotted on the scattergram of the two variables simply by adding the line

$$0.001\,948 \times \text{BIRTHWEIGHT} - 16.0846 \times \text{FACTOR68} - 0.5036 = 0 \quad (10.8)$$

This is shown in Figure 10.2. A new infant with a position above the line would be allocated to the SIDS group, and below the line to the control group. Boxplots of the discriminant function scores for cases and controls are shown in Figure 10.3.

A deficiency of the allocation rule derived above is that it takes no account of the *prior probability* of class membership in the population under study. So if used in this simple form as a screening device for babies at risk of SIDS, many more infants would be considered at risk than is genuinely merited, since SIDS is known to be a relatively rare condition. To accommodate prior probabilities into the rule, it must be adjusted to the following

Assign subject to group one if $z_i - z_c > \ln Q$
Assign subject to group two if $z_i - z_c \leqslant \ln Q$

where

$$Q = \frac{\text{Prior probability of group one}}{\text{Prior probability of group two}} \quad (10.9)$$

Prior probabilities are often ignored in published accounts of the application of discriminant function analysis, the implicit assumption then being made that $P(\text{Group one}) = P(\text{Group two}) = 0.5$.

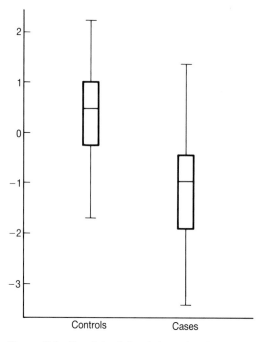

Figure 10.3   Boxplots of discriminant function scores for SIDS data

A question of some importance about a discriminant function is 'how well does it perform?' An obvious method of evaluating performance would be to apply the derived classification rule to the original data and assess the misclassification rate. Table 10.3 shows the results of this procedure for the SIDS data. The misclassification rate of 17% is quite low, but estimated in this way using the original data, is known generally to be an optimistic estimator of the actual misclassification rate. A more realistic estimate of the latter may be obtained in a variety of ways (see Hand, 1986, for details). Perhaps the most straightforward of these is the so-called 'leaving one out method', where the discriminant function is derived on the basis of $n - 1$ of the individuals under consideration and then used to classify the individual not included. The whole process is repeated, each time omitting a different individual. Applying this procedure to the SIDS data gives the results shown in Table 10.4. The estimated misclassification rate rises a little to 19%. In many applications, the difference between the two estimates will be much greater.

The discriminant function derived above makes the assumption that the two populations of interest have the same covariance matrix. If this is not the case a linear discriminant function is no longer suitable for separating the two groups. A more complex *quadratic discriminant function* is needed — see Everitt and Dunn (1991) for details.

The equality of covariance matrices was the only assumption made by Fisher in the original derivation of the linear discriminant function. It can be shown however that the method is optimal *only* if the two populations have

Table 10.3 Classification matrix for Fisher's discriminant function for SIDS data using BIRTHWEIGHT and FACTOR68

Group	Percent correct	Number of cases classified into group	
		Controls	Cases
Controls	83.7	41	8
Cases	81.3	3	13
Total	83.1	44	21

Table 10.4 Jack-knifed classification for SIDS data

Group	Percent correct	Number of cases classified into group	
		Controls	Cases
Controls	81.6	40	9
Cases	81.3	3	13
Total	81.5	43	22

multivariate normal distributions. In particular when some of the observed variables are, for example, binary, Fisher's linear discriminant function may not be the most suitable assignment technique to use, a point taken up further in Section 10.3.

Returning to the SIDS data, the linear discriminant function for all four variables can be found from the mean vectors and within-group covariance matrix given in Table 10.5 by once again applying (10.2). The result is as follows

$$z = 0.001\,79 \times \text{BIRTHWEIGHT} - 15.533 \times \text{FACTOR68}$$
$$- 0.001\,78 \times \text{HEARTRATE} + 0.215 \times \text{GESAGE} \qquad (10.10)$$

In practical applications of the linear discriminant functions one of the most important requirements is often to select a subset of the available variables, which can can be considered to be the best discriminators. (Compare selecting variables in regression analysis — see Chapter 5.) In general, stepwise procedures similar to those that have been described in Chapters 5 and 8 are used. The criteria for entering and removing variables are the same as those used in multiple regression — see Chapter 5. Applying the procedure to all four variables in the SIDS data gives the results shown in Table 10.6. Clearly BIRTHWEIGHT and the FACTOR68 variable are the two variables which discriminate most successfully between the cases and controls in this example.

It is of some interest to note that it is possible to obtain the coefficients defining the linear discriminant function by using a regression approach. A dummy variable, y, is introduced which takes on a different value for members of group one and group two. If the two data sets are then treated as a single

Table 10.5　Means and pooled covariance matrix for all variables in SIDS data

Means

Variable	Controls	Cases
BIRTHWEIGHT	3437.86	2964.69
FACTOR68	0.31	0.40
HEARTRATE	129.24	132.95
GESAGE	40.00	39.25

Covariance matrix

	1	2	3	4
BIRTHWEIGHT	278612.28			
FACTOR68	4.32	0.0062		
HEARTRATE	130.94	0.24	269.40	
GESAGE	196.29	−0.01	1.26	1.09

Table 10.6　Results of stepwise selection procedure for Fisher's discriminant function on SIDS data

Step 0

Variable	F to enter d.f. = 1 and 63
BIRTHWEIGHT	9.69
FACTOR68	16.15
HEARTRATE	0.62
GESAGE	6.19

Step 1

Variable entered FACTOR68

Variable	F to enter d.f. 1 and 62
BIRTHWEIGHT	9.88
HEARTRATE	0.00
GESAGE	3.08

Step 2

Variable entered BIRTHWEIGHT

Variable	F to enter d.f. 1 and 61
HEARTRATE	0.00
GESAGE	0.33

No more variables entered

sample of size $n_1 + n_2$, the coefficients in the regression of y on $x_1, x_2, \ldots, x_p$, are proportional to $\mathbf{S}^{-1}(\bar{\mathbf{x}}_1 - \bar{\mathbf{x}}_2)$. Any two values could be used to identify group membership but the most convenient are $n_2/(n_1 + n_2)$ for observations from group one and $-n_1/(n_1 + n_2)$ for observations from group two. The average of the dummy variable over the whole data is now zero, and a new individual is allocated to group one or group two according to whether the corresponding predicted value of y is positive or negative.

When more than two groups are involved, Fisher's linear discriminant method as described above can be extended relatively simply to provide an appropriate classification rule. With three groups, for example, the rule would be based on three functions.

$$h_{12}(\mathbf{x}) = (\bar{\mathbf{x}}_1 - \bar{\mathbf{x}}_2)'\mathbf{S}^{-1}[\mathbf{x} - \tfrac{1}{2}(\bar{\mathbf{x}}_1 + \bar{\mathbf{x}}_2)] \qquad (10.11)$$

$$h_{13}(\mathbf{x}) = (\bar{\mathbf{x}}_1 - \bar{\mathbf{x}}_3)'\mathbf{S}^{-1}[\mathbf{x} - \tfrac{1}{2}(\bar{\mathbf{x}}_1 + \bar{\mathbf{x}}_3)] \qquad (10.12)$$

$$h_{23}(\mathbf{x}) = (\bar{\mathbf{x}}_2 - \bar{\mathbf{x}}_3)'\mathbf{S}^{-1}[\mathbf{x} - \tfrac{1}{2}(\bar{\mathbf{x}}_2 + \bar{\mathbf{x}}_3)] \qquad (10.13)$$

The classification rule now becomes: allocate an individual with vector of observations, $\mathbf{x}$ to

Group one if $h_{12}(\mathbf{x}) > 0$ and $h_{13}(\mathbf{x}) > 0$
Group two if $h_{12}(\mathbf{x}) < 0$ and $h_{23}(\mathbf{x}) > 0$
Group three if $h_{13}(\mathbf{x}) < 0$ and $h_{23}(\mathbf{x}) < 0$

As mentioned previously, Fisher's linear discriminant function is optimal when the two populations have multivariate normal densities with equal covariance matrices, although it has been shown to be relatively robust to departures from normality (see, for example, Gilbert, 1968, Moore, 1973 and Krzanowski, 1977). In some cases, however, when the normality assumption is clearly invalid, an alternative allocation method should be considered. One used widely in medical investigations is based on the logistic regression model met previously in Chapter 5.

10.3 Logistic discrimination

The essential feature of this approach to discrimination is to assume the following form for the probabilities of class membership (only the two group situation will be considered here).

$$P(\text{Group one}) = \exp\left(\beta_0 + \sum_{i=1}^{p}\beta_i x_i\right)\Big/\left[1 + \exp\left(\beta_0 + \sum_{i=1}^{p}\beta_i x_i\right)\right] \qquad (10.14)$$

$$P(\text{Group two}) = 1\Big/\left[1 + \exp\left(\beta_0 + \sum_{i=1}^{p}\beta_i x_i\right)\right] \qquad (10.15)$$

The parameters $\beta_0, \beta_1, \ldots, \beta_p$ may be estimated by maximum likelihood methods (see Anderson, 1972). The important point is that the estimation process is *independent* of the form assumed for the class density functions. Day and Kerridge (1967) and Anderson (1972) show that this method of discrimination has optimal properties under a wide range of assumptions about the underlying distributions, including those relevant when both continuous and categorical variable are used to describe each individual.

After estimation of the parameters, allocation of new individuals can be performed on the basis of scores given by

$$\hat{\beta}_0 + \sum_{i=1}^{p}\hat{\beta}_i x_i \qquad (10.16)$$

If this is positive the individual is allocated to group one (since P (group

174 *Assignment Techniques*

Table 10.7 Enuresis data

Treatment Group	x_1	x_2	x_3	x_4	x_5
1	0	0	8.4	1	0
1	1	0	8.7	1	0
1	0	0	8.9	1	1
1	1	0	8.1	1	1
1	1	0	8.6	1	0
1	1	0	8.9	1	0
1	1	0	8.5	0	0
1	1	0	6.3	1	0
1	0	0	5.3	1	0
1	1	0	8.7	0	0
1	0	0	8.6	1	0
1	1	0	9.0	1	0
1	1	0	8.3	1	1
1	1	0	8.1	1	0
1	1	1	8.5	1	1
1	0	0	7.6	1	0
1	1	0	4.3	1	0
1	1	0	6.8	1	0
1	0	0	5.9	1	0
1	1	0	8.7	1	0
1	1	0	5.9	1	0
1	0	0	9.0	1	0
1	0	0	8.4	1	0
1	0	0	8.2	1	0
1	1	0	8.6	1	1
1	1	0	6.4	0	1
2	0	0	8.1	1	0
2	1	0	8.6	1	0
2	0	0	8.2	1	0
2	0	0	8.8	0	0
2	0	0	8.1	1	0
2	0	0	8.5	1	0
2	1	0	8.9	1	0
2	1	0	8.1	1	0
2	0	0	5.3	1	0
2	0	0	4.8	1	0
2	0	0	5.1	1	0
2	1	0	8.4	1	0
2	0	0	9.0	0	0
2	1	0	8.7	0	0
2	0	0	4.6	1	0
2	0	0	6.7	1	0
2	0	0	8.1	1	1
2	1	0	7.4	1	0
2	1	0	7.1	1	0
2	1	0	6.4	1	0
2	0	1	7.8	1	0
2	1	0	8.7	1	1
2	0	0	9.1	1	0
2	0	0	8.4	1	0

x_1 = Whether or not there were family background difficulties (1 = yes, 0 = no)
x_2 = Whether wetting occured during the day (1 = yes, 0 = no)
x_3 = Child's age (years)
x_4 = Whether family had access to an inside w.c. (1 = yes, 0 = no)
x_5 = Whether the child shared a room with more than one sibling (1 = yes, 0 = no)

Table 10.8 Parameter estimates and standard errors for logistic discrimination on enuresis data

Variable	Coefficient	SE	Coeff/SE
FBGD	1.049	0.610	1.72
WET	−0.4879	1.68	−0.291
WC	0.3380	0.946	0.357
SHARE	0.9895	0.926	1.07
AGE	0.034	0.230	0.148
CONSTANT	−1.147	2.12	−0.541

one) > P (group two)), if negative to group two. Thus when the logistic form is assumed for the probabilities of group membership, the result is again a linear discriminant function. (This rule assumes equal prior probabilities for the two groups.)

To illustrate the application of logistic discrimination in practice it will be applied to the data shown in Table 10.7, adapted from Hand (1981). These data were collected in a study designed to investigate whether the outcome of treating enuretic children with an alarm buzzer could be predicted from certain observations made on the children. The two groups involved were:

Group 1 — failure or relapse after apparent cure,
Group 2 — long term cure.

The estimates of the parameters and their standard errors are shown in Table 10.8. Using these estimates the allocation rule becomes: allocate a child with scores $x_1, x_2, \ldots, x_5$ to group one if

$$1.049x_1 - 0.4879x_2 + 0.330x_3 + 0.9895x_4 + 0.034402x_5 - 1.147 > 0 \quad (10.17)$$

The performance of the rule may again be assessed (albeit optimistically) by comparing actual and predicted groupings on the original data. The misclassifciation rate is 36%. Applying Fisher's method to these data gives the following classification rule for allocating a child to group one

$$1.073x_1 - 0.445x_2 + 0.328x_3 + 0.908x_4 + 0.034x_5 - 1.235 > 0 \quad (10.18)$$

very similar to the rule given in (10.17).

Choosing a small subset of variables which discriminate adequately when applying logistic discrimination is again undertaken by some form of stepwise procedure, the relevant criterion used being the difference in the values of a chi-square statistic. For the enuresis data such a procedure leads to selecting only the family background difficulties variable. The corresponding allocation rule now becomes very simple; if a child is considered to have family background difficulties it seems that the treatment with an alarm buzzer is likely to fail.

10.4 Computer-assisted diagnosis

Since the mid 1970s a great deal of research effort has been devoted to the development of sophisticated methodologies able to cope with complex

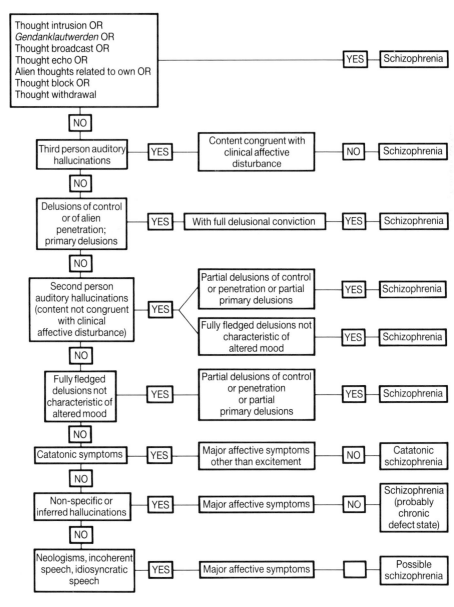

Figure 10.4   A flowchart for the diagnosis of schizophrenia

problems such as medical decision making. One of the main aims of such systems is to assist the physician in the process of diagnosis, a procedure defined by the *Concise Oxford Dictionary* as, the 'identification of disease by means of a patient's symptoms etc'. Clearly the assignment techniques described earlier constitute one approach to assisting clinicians in their diagnostic role. A number of other methods are available, however, particularly those based

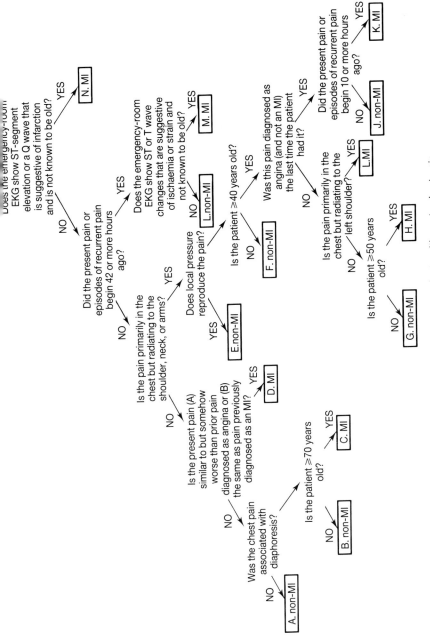

Figure 10.5 Computer derived decision tree for the classification of patients with acute chest pain

on hierarchical flowcharts. An example will best serve to illustrate this type of approach and Figure 10.4 presents an illustration of flowchart ideas applied to the diagnosis of schizophrenia. The diagram represents a hierarchical way of classifying the current mental state of patients, which would probably be roughly in agreement with the views of the majority of British psychiatrists. This type of flowchart is referred to by Hand (1985) as *mechanistic* since the questions and branch points are derived from clinical expertise, rather than from a statistical appraisal of a suitable database. Empirical flowcharts arise when the branching structure of the decision tree is derived from objective mathematical and statistical methods, perhaps using a previously created database. An example of such a flowchart is that derived by Goldman *et al.* (1982) for assisting in the diagnosis of myocardial infarction. These workers began with a large number of variables and examined them one by one to identify the particular variable which best separated the infarction and non-infarction groups, 'best separation' being defined in a particular way which involved consideration of the 'cost' of misclassification (readers are referred to the original paper for details). Splitting the patients into two groups using the chosen variable yields groups containing predominantly infarction cases and non-infarction cases. Each of these two groups is then examined separately, searching for the variable which best discriminates between the two diagnostic categories within the group. This was repeated until sufficient accuracy was achieved. The resulting flowchart is shown in Figure 10.5

Other examples of empirically derived flowcharts for diagnosis are given in Feldman *et al.* (1972) and Sturt (1981).

10.5 Summary

Discriminant analysis techniques produce rules which can be used to classify new individuals for whom the true classification may not be known. There are many different techniques which might be used and an excellent overview is provided by Hand (1981, 1992) who also describes a number of fascinating examples of the use of assignment techniques in a medical context. In this chapter the two most commonly used methods, Fisher's linear discriminant function and logistic discrimination, have been described. The former is optimal when the classes have multivariate normal densities with the same covariance matrix, and the latter is applicable to a wide range of class density functions. Other methods which can be used as aids in the diagnostic process are those based on hierarchical flowcharts. Such charts, although often very useful, are sometimes regarded as too rigid, fixed or predetermined, and much recent research effort has been devoted to the development of expert systems for diagnosis which are flexible and able to respond to any input datum in sensible manner. One such system is described by Shortliffe (1976) and an introductory overview is provided in Hand (1985).

11

The Analysis of Time Series

11.1 Introduction

A *time series* is a sequence of numerical data in which each value is associated with a particular instant in time. Such data arise frequently in medical investigations, for example: weekly entries into a hospital, monthly mortality rates for a particular disease, or annual deaths from say cancer. In most (but not all) series the variable of interest is continuous and is recorded at a discrete set of time points, generally equally spaced, at least approximately. Series with unequally spaced values are more difficult to deal with and will not be considered in this chapter. The observations in a series will be denoted by $x_1, x_2, \ldots, x_n$ where n is the length of the series.

It might be thought that the statistical method appropriate for examining and analysing time series data would be some type of regression, with the measurement made at each time point being the dependent variable and time the explanatory variable. The regression models described in Chapter 5 are, however, unlikely to be particularly helpful for a number of reasons. First, the patterns exhibited by time series data are generally far more complex then could be accommodated by such models. Second, the observations in a time series are very unlikely to be independent of one another. Neighbouring observations are frequently positively correlated, with the correlation becoming stronger as the time interval between them becomes shorter. In a series of hourly blood pressure readings, for example, a 'high' reading at one o'clock is likely to have a certain inertia and remain high at two o'clock. The existence of a possibly complex pattern of dependence between observations in different parts of a time series, implies that methods of analysis which assume that the observations are independent will not be appropriate. Consequently special methods of analysis have been developed for time series data and several of these will be briefly described in this chapter. For a more detailed account of the methods, particularly the theory behind them, readers are referred to Chatfield (1989).

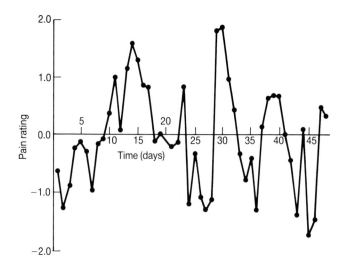

Figure 11.1   Migraine headache patient's ratings of severity of his headache pain

11.2 Preliminary analysis of time series

Many time series can be considered to be a mixture of four components:

(1)   a *trend* or long term movement,
(2)   fluctuations about the trend of greater or lesser regularity,
(3)   a deterministic cycle, for example, a pronounced seasonal component,
(4)   a residual, irregular or random effect.

The aims of a time series analysis are not usually so clear cut as, for example, in fitting a regression model. Part of the analysis may seek to provide a description of regular or systematic variation, for example by identifying periodic effects or cycles. Additionally it might be hoped to develop models for the series which allow inferences about the mechanisms generating the series and the possibility of making predictions about future values of the series. The essential *first* step in the analysis of any time series, however, should be simply to plot the observations against time. Figure 11.1, for example, shows the daily ratings of headache pain given by a migraine sufferer, and Figure 11.2 the number of deaths per quarter from ischaemic heart disease suffered by males in the U.K. The data leading to Figure 11.2 (taken from Dunstan, 1993), are given in Table 11.1. Such plots are often valuable in highlighting qualitative features such as, for example, a trend, seasonality or outliers, although such patterns are frequently obscured by 'noise' making them extremely difficult to detect without more formal analyses. (Some examples that illustrate this latter point will be given later.) On the other hand it should not be overlooked that a simple plot of the data can often suggest patterns in the data which, on further investigation, are found to be illusory.

After plotting the series, the first and simplest hypothesis that might be considered is that it is random. (A so called *white noise series*.) A number

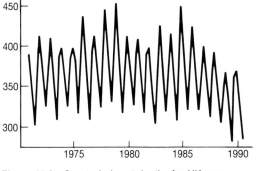

Figure 11.2 Quarterly heart deaths for UK men

Table 11.1 Quarterly deaths from heart disease for males in the UK – 1967 to 1991

389	345	303	362	412	356	325	375
410	350	310	388	399	362	325	382
399	382	318	385	437	357	310	391
413	377	325	381	446	382	331	387
454	370	318	372	412	370	327	386
408	361	318	390	399	340	305	369
427	364	321	371	415	373	309	370
450	369	321	368	424	363	321	353
400	343	312	368	392	340	305	347
367	335	282	362	369	323	287	

of formal tests of such a hypothesis that are available are described in detail in Kendall and Ord (1990). In general, however, such tests are not of great importance in respect of the original series since in most instances this will clearly be non-random. Tests of randomness assume greater importance once an attempt has been made to extract the systematic components of a series and residuals are examined for evidence of any remaining regularities.

11.3 Transforming a series to stationarity

Often the first formal step in the analysis of a time series is to examine how it might be transformed to *stationarity*. Stationary series have the characteristics that a graph of the series against time looks qualitatively about the same near one time interval as near another. An explicit definition is that all statistical properties of such series remain unchanged when the period of observation is moved forward or backward in time. In particular the mean and variance of a stationary time series do not change with time. Furthermore the *autocovariance* (see later), between values of the series separated by a particular number of time points, depends only on the time difference or *lag*, not on the time instance. Transformation to stationarity is usually a necessary prerequisite to exploring series with a view to fitting the types of model to be described later in this chapter.

Departures from stationarity have several possible causes. Many series are not stationary because of the presence of a trend, see for example Figure 11.3. This feature of a series needs to be described and estimated in some way so that it can be removed before the series is analysed further. One approach would be to estimate the trend component by least squares fitting of a straight line or perhaps some low degree polynomial, and then subtract the estimated values from those in the original series. An alternate possibility is to estimate the trend by a simple *moving average*, calculated as follows

$$u_t = \frac{1}{2q+1} \sum_{i=t-q}^{i=t+q} x_i \tag{11.1}$$

A widely used method which does not estimate the trend directly, but removes it to try to produce a stationary series, is based on *differencing*. A linear trend, for example, can be removed by simply calculating first differences

$$u_t = x_t - x_{t-1} \tag{11.2}$$

If there is a quadratic trend in a series, then the values of the first differences should be reduced to having a linear trend. Applying the method again, to calculate the second differences, should remove the quadratic trend altogether. So in this case, first differences of the series of first differences, u_t, created by (11.2) would be calculated

$$y_t = u_t - u_{t-1} = x_t - 2x_{t-1} + x_{t-2} \tag{11.3}$$

Time series are often non-stationary because of the presence of periodicities such as those caused by a seasonal cycle, and the differencing technique can again be used to remove such components from a series. In a monthly series with annual periodicity, for example, differences between values in corresponding months would be calculated

$$u_t = x_t - x_{t-12} \tag{11.4}$$

If a series contains both trend and seasonal effects then both can be removed by combining both types of differencing operation. To illustrate the technique consider again the deaths from heart disease data given in Table 11.1. The plot of these data (Figure 11.2), shows a very clear periodic component of an annual nature. There is also some evidence of a quadratic trend with number of deaths declining towards the end of the period of recording. So taking first, second differences, gives the results shown in Figure 11.4. The new series shows no trend component although the annual cycle is still very evident. Applying next the transformation.

$$u_t = x_t - x_{t-4} \tag{11.5}$$

leads to the series shows in Figure 11.5. This series contains no obvious trend or periodic components, and the two differencing procedures have together produced a seemingly stationary series.

In some circumstances it may be appropriate to take some simple transformation of the original series before attempting to remove trend and/or

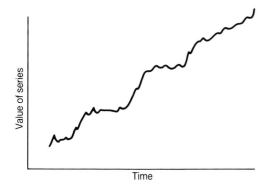

Figure 11.3   Time series with a clear trend

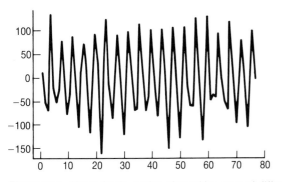

Figure 11.4   Heart deaths series after taking second differences

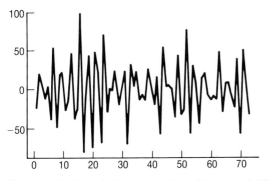

Figure 11.5   Heart deaths series after taking second differences and removing seasonal effect

seasonal effects. If, for example, it is found that the variance is related to the mean, then a variance-stabilizing transformation should be applied. Figure 11.6, for example, shows a series with clear trend and periodic components, with the seasonal effect growing in magnitude as the overall mean increases. Here, the differencing operations considered previously, if simply applied to the raw data, would not necessarily remove both trend and cyclic component.

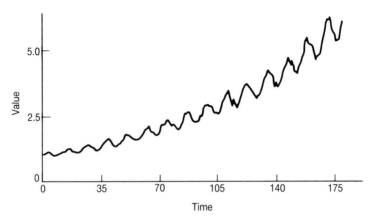

Figure 11.6   Time series with trend and periodic components and changing variance

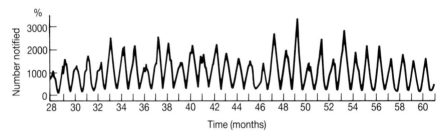

Figure 11.7   Monthly notifications of chicken-pox for New York City from 1928 to 1960

Helfenstein (1986) suggests that a practical tool for choosing the appropriate transformation from a class defined by

$$x_t^{(\lambda)} = x_t^{\lambda}, \lambda \neq 0 \text{ (power transformation)} \tag{11.6}$$
$$= \ln x_t, \lambda = 0 \text{ (logarithmic transformation)} \tag{11.7}$$

is the *mean-range* plot, in which the range is plotted against the mean for each seasonal period. If the range is independent of the mean, no transformation is needed ($\lambda = 1$). If the plot displays random scatter about a straight line, the logarithmic transformation is appropriate ($\lambda = 0$). To illustrate his suggested procedure, Helfenstein uses a series giving monthly notifications of chicken-pox in New York City from 1928 to 1960. The series is plotted in Figure 11.7. The mean-range plot for the data is shown in Figure 11.8(a). The points appear to scatter around a straight line, suggesting that a logarithmic transformation should be applied. The mean-range plot for the log-transformed series shown in Figure 11.8(b), appears to confirm that such a transformation is appropriate. The log transformed series is shown in Figure 11.9 and again in Figure 11.10 *after* the removal of the seasonal effect by differencing.

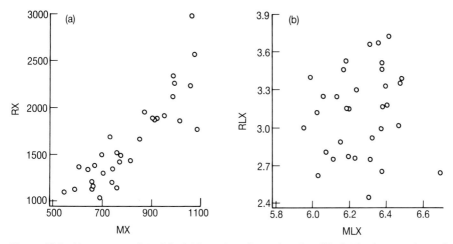

Figure 11.8 Mean-range plots: (a) plot for untransformed series, (b) plot for log transformed series.

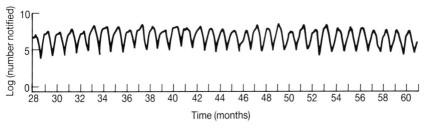

Figure 11.9 Log transformed chicken-pox data

11.4 Analysing time series: (1) frequency domain methods

Modern methods for the analysis of time series data can be divided roughly into two classes — *frequency domain* methods and *time domain* methods. The latter are based on direct modelling of the lagged relationships between a series and its past and are the subject of Section 11.5. The primary aim of frequency domain methods for the analysis of time series is to identify oscillations of major importance, in the sense of explaining a large proportion of the variance

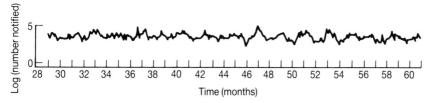

Figure 11.10 Log transformed chicken-pox data after removal of seasonal effect

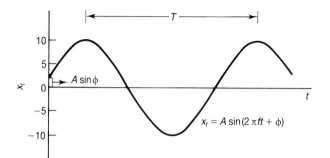

Figure 11.11   Example of a sine wave with amplitude A, frequency f, period T and phase ϕ

in an observed series. Methods in this class are derived from the earlier ideas of Fourier analysis, in which a series of observations is represented as a superposition of independently varying cosine and sine curves. A typical sine wave, for example, has the form

$$x_t = A \sin(2\pi f t + \phi) \tag{11.8}$$

where the constant, A, is called the *amplitude*, f the *frequency* and ϕ the *phase*. The curve is *periodic* with a period, $T = 1/f$. This simply means that the plot of x_t against t is the same at $t + 1/f, t + 2/f, \ldots$ etc., as at t. An example of a sine wave is shown in Figure 11.11.

An early tool for the analysis of time series data which used the idea of Fourier decomposition was the *Schuster periodogram*. (Schuster, 1898). Observations on the time series are expressed exactly as a superposition of cosine curves of the form

$$x_t = A_0 + \sum_{k=1}^{(n-1)/2} A_k \cos(2\pi f_k t + \phi_k) \tag{11.9}$$

The amplitudes, A_k, and phases, ϕ_k can be calculated from the data, with A_k indicating the importance of oscillations of period $1/f_k$ in the observed series. The periodogram is the graph of nA_k^2 against k. If the original series contains an exact cyclic component with a particular period, then the periodogram can be expected to have a sharp peak at the appropriate value of k. Figure 11.12 for example, shows the periodogram of the heart deaths data (Table 11.1). There is a clear peak corresponding to the annual cycle.

In practice however, the periodogram is of little use since the values, A_k, usually have great statistical variability and the plot is usually extremely irregular. Apparent peaks are easy to find, even in the absence of genuine cycles, because one or more local maxima will often appear substantially larger than neighbouring values.

Most current frequency domain analysis techniques are less concerned with the discovery of exact periodicities and more concerned with estimating the *spectral density* or *spectrum* of the series, this being a function, $S(f)$, of the frequency, f, that summarizes how the variance of the series is distributed amongst oscillations of different frequencies. Usually estimation of the spec-

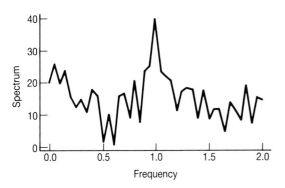

Figure 11.12 Periodogram of deaths from heart disease series

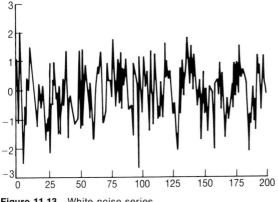

Figure 11.13 White noise series

trum is approached non-parametrically, without assuming a particular form for $S(f)$. Details can be found in Jenkins and Watts (1968).

The spectrum of a white noise series is constant (flat). Here there is absolutely no regularity and all cycles are present with equal intensity, much as white light consists of light of all colours mixed with equal brightness. Figure 11.13 shows an example of such a series.

Systematic structure in a time series is indicated by a departure from flatness in the spectrum. A peak in $S(f)$ suggests that the series has a tendency to cycle at a particular frequency. As an illustration consider the series shown in Figure 11.14; this series consists of a pure sine wave process masked by white noise. It is extremely difficult to detect any pure cycle in Figure 11.14. The estimated spectral density shown in Figure 11.15, however, shows a sharp peak at exactly the frequency of the hidden cycle. Clearly a spectral analysis of a time series can point out structure in the data not visible in a simple plot of the series.

Spectral analysis has been widely used in the analysis of EEG recordings and a review is given in Dumermuth *et al.* (1976). An interesting application

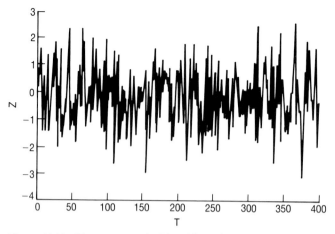

Figure 11.14   Sine wave masked by white noise

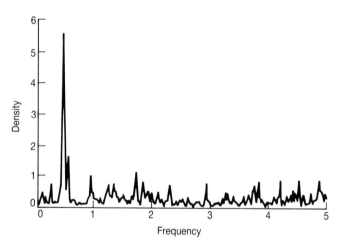

Figure 11.15   Spectral density of a sine wave masked by white noise

discussed by Bosaeus *et al.* (1977) involves the use of the spectra of EEG recordings to discriminate between normal children and children with minimal brain dysfunction.

11.5 Analysing time series: (2) time domain methods

The models to be described later in this section are designed to aid investigators dealing with time series data, particularly in the following three situations.

(1) Epidemilogists are often faced with assessing the relationship between a target or output series, such as daily number of patients coming to a clinic

and explanatory or input series such as daily concentration of a pollutant. Important here are the so called *transfer function models*.
(2) Questions about changes in time series are frequently of great importance in medicine. An investigator might, for example, be interested in assessing how the pattern of morbidity in a population changes after an environmental accident, or in measuring the effectiveness of a campaign to make teenagers aware of the dangers of AIDS. Such questions can be investigated by the *intervention analysis* methods proposed originally by Box and Tiao (1975).
(3) Accurate forecasts of the future values of a time series may be of great value in many areas of medicine. Public health organizations, for example, need to know what frequencies of diseases might be expected in coming years in order to plan how to allocate often limited resources.

The *Box–Jenkins* models to be discussed later are fundamental for all three situations.

An important initial step in the search for an appropriate model for a time series is an examination of the dependence structure of the series. The basic tool in this process is the *correlogram*.

11.5.1 The correlogram

After plotting the raw data, identifying and extracting trend and seasonal components, the next stage in the analysis of a time series is to calculate the *autocovariance* or *autocorrelation* function of the series. These both arise from considering pairs of observations separated by different time intervals. Given the series, $x_1, x_2, \ldots, x_n$, for example, the $n-1$ pairs $(x_1, x_2), (x_1, x_3), \ldots, (x_{n-1}, x_n)$, constitute a set of bivariate values for which a covariance or correlation may be calculated. Similarly, for the $n-2$ pairs, $(x_1, x_3), (x_2, x_4), \ldots, (x_{n-2}, x_n)$ and so on. A plot of the values of these correlations against the particular time lag involved is known as a *correlogram*. Mathematically, the autocovariance and autocorrelation of lag k are defined as follows:

$$\text{autocovariance}(k) = \frac{1}{n} \sum_{i=1}^{n-k} (x_t - \bar{x})(x_{t+k} - \bar{x}) \qquad (11.10)$$

where $\bar{x} = \frac{1}{n} \sum_{i=1}^{n} x_i$ is the mean of the series

$$\text{autocorrelation}(k) = \frac{\text{autocovariance}(k)}{\text{autocovariance}(0)} \qquad (11.11)$$

The correlogram is very useful for distinguishing between different types of series and for choosing appropriate models. To interpret the correlogram it is necessary to know how large values must be, to be regarded as important. As with ordinary correlation coefficients values of autocorrelations must lie between -1 and $+1$, with values near these extremes indicating a high degree of linear dependence. Values close to zero suggest that the corresponding observations are independent. Approximate 95% confidence limits for the values of the autocorrelation for a series of n independent observations are $-2/\sqrt{n}$ and $2/\sqrt{n}$. If a series has almost all the values in the autocorrelation function

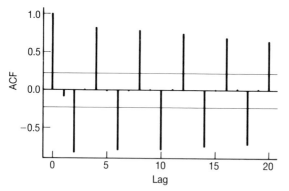

Figure 11.16   Correlogram for second differenced heart deaths data

within these limits, then the observations can be regarded as independent. The lags corresponding to autocorrelations outside the limits are generally useful in indicating which type of model is appropriate for the series, as will be seen later.

It is important to remember that the correlogram is really only useful for suggesting possible models, after trend and cyclic components have been removed from the series. The structure of the correlogram for non-stationary series will usually only reflect the source of the non-stationarity. A trend in a time series, for example, will lead to a correlogram in which the correlations will not come down to zero except for very large values of the lag. If a time series contains seasonal fluctuations, then the correlogram will also exhibit an oscillation of the same frequency. With a quarterly series for example, the autocorrelation of lag two will be 'large' and negative, whilst that for lag four will be 'large' and positive with subsequent correlations showing the same pattern. This is clearly demonstrated in Figure 11.16 which shown the correlogram for the second differenced heart disease deaths data. The sinusoidal pattern of the correlogram is very evident, but provides little extra information as the seasonal pattern is obvious in the time plot of the data.

The correlogram of the heart disease deaths data, *after* removal of both trend and seasonal components by differencing as described earlier, is shown in Figure 11.17. Now the autocorrelations beyond lag four do not differ significantly from zero. This 'dampening' of the correlations as the lag increases is a characteristic of series well described by a particular type of model as will be seen later.

(Both correlogram and spectrum, which are essentially equivalent descriptions of a series, are very useful in suggesting what types of model might account for the data, or perhaps equally usefully, in dismissing some models as inadequate.)

11.5.2 Models for time series

Time series data are most often modelled by *autoregressive* models or by a combination of autoregressive and *moving average* models. Autoregressive models express the observation, x_t, as a linear function of the past values of

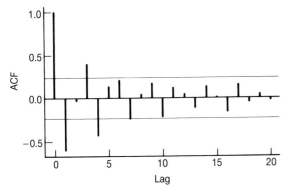

Figure 11.17 Correlogram of heart deaths data after taking second differences and after removal of seasonal effect

the series. The simplest example of such a model is

$$x_t = \phi x_{t-1} + \epsilon_t \qquad (11.12)$$

which is known as a *first order autoregressive model*. The parameter ϕ must be estimated from the values of the series, and the ϵ_t are a series of independent, identically distributed random variables whose distribution is approximately normal with mean zero and variance σ^2. The general autoregressive model of order p has the form

$$x_t = \phi_1 x_{t-1} + \phi_2 x_{t-2} + \ldots + \phi_p x_{t-p} + \epsilon_t \qquad (11.13)$$

This model expresses the current observation as a linear combination of past observations plus a residual disturbance term, ϵ_t, usually regarded as white noise. In many instances, however, there is evidence that although the series has some features characteristic of an autoregressive model, the ϵ_t are *not* white noise, but are themselves correlated. A plausible model for the disturbances is that they are produced by a superposition of lagged white noise terms leading to the so called moving average model of order q given by

$$\epsilon_t = a_t + \theta_1 a_{t-1} + \theta_2 a_{t-2} + \ldots, \theta_q a_{t-q} \qquad (11.14)$$

where a_t is a white noise series and $\theta_1, \theta_2, \ldots, \theta_q$ are parameters to be estimated.
The combination of these two models, that is

$$x_t = \phi_1 x_{t-1} + \phi_2 x_{t_2} + \ldots + \phi_p x_{t-p} + a_t + \theta_1 a_{t-1} + \theta_2 a_{t-2} + \ldots + \theta_q a_{t-q} \quad (11.15)$$

is referred to as an *autoregressive moving average* model of order p and q, usually abbreviated to ARMA (p, q). Many *stationary series* can be described by ARMA models with relatively small values of p and q. The coefficients in the models may be estimated by a variety of techniques including maximum likelihood and non-linear least squares. Possible values for p and q are generally gleaned from studying the correlogram. An autoregressive model of order one, for example, has a correlogram in which the correlations gradually die away as the lag increases. A moving average process of order one, however, has a correlogram in which all the correlations for lags greater than one are zero.
The model in (11.15) is expressed in terms of a stationary series obtained

Table 11.2   Results from fitting a series of ARIMA models to heart deaths data

---

(1) ARIMA(1,2,0)
$\hat{\phi}_1 = -0.62$, SE $= 0.09$.
(2) ARIMA(0,2,1)
$\hat{\theta}_1 = 1.00$, SE $= 0.003$.
(3) ARIMA(1,2,1)
$\hat{\phi}_1 = -0.46$, SE $= 0.11$.
$\hat{\theta}_1 = 1.00$, SE $= 0.005$.
(4) ARIMA(1,2,2)
$\hat{\phi} = 0.07$, SE $= 0.12$.
$\hat{\theta}_1 = 1.98, \hat{\theta}_2 = -0.98$, SE$(\hat{\theta}_1) = 0.022$, SE$(\hat{\theta}_2) = 0.022$.

---

after some type of differencing operation. In terms of the original series the model is said to be an *autoregressive integrated moving average* process, abbreviated to ARIMA (p, d, q). The extra term, *d*, refers to the amount of differencing necessary to achieve stationarity. (The model can be expanded further to incorporate possible seasonal effects directly, but this will not be considered here; see Dunstan, 1993, for a readable account with examples.)

To illustrate the use of ARIMA models, the heart disease deaths series will be used, after applying the differencing operation (11.4), to remove the seasonal component. (Note that here second differences to remove the possible quadratic trend will *not* be applied directly but will be incorporated into the fitted ARIMA model by using the appropriate value of *d*.) The results of fitting a series of models with different values of *p* and *q* but all with the value $d = 2$ are shown in Table 11.2. Various criteria are available for choosing between models (for details see Dunstan, 1993). Here plots of the standardized residuals and the correlogram of these residuals will be examined. The plots for the simple first order autoregressive model (ARIMA (1, 2, 0)) are shown in Figures 11.18 (a) and 11.18 (b). There are some large residuals and a number of the autocorrelations are greater than zero. Both findings suggest that this model does not fit the data very well. Similar comments apply to the simple first order moving average model (ARIMA (0, 2,1)) — see Figures 11.19 (a) and 11.19 (b). The residuals from fitting an ARIMA (1, 2, 1) model are shown in Figure 11.20 (a). Again some of these are rather large, although the correlogram of the residuals (Figure 11.20 (b)) shows that all but one of the autocorrelations are zero. Finally the results from an ARIMA (1, 2, 2) model appear in Figure 11.21. One or two of the residuals from this model remain rather large, but their autocorrelations all full within the 95% confidence limits. This model seems to provide a reasonable fit for the series and could perhaps be used as the basis for forecasting (see Dunstan, 1993).

11.6 Summary

The analysis of time series is a large and complex area. In this chapter brief accounts only have been given of the main techniques such as spectral analysis

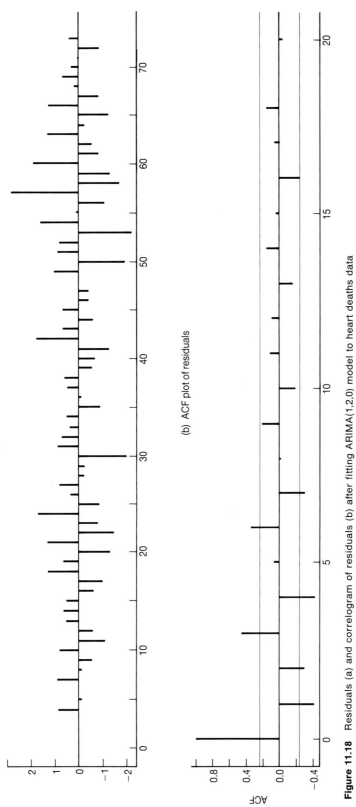

(a) Plot of standardized residuals

(b) ACF plot of residuals

Figure 11.18 Residuals (a) and correlogram of residuals (b) after fitting ARIMA(1,2,0) model to heart deaths data

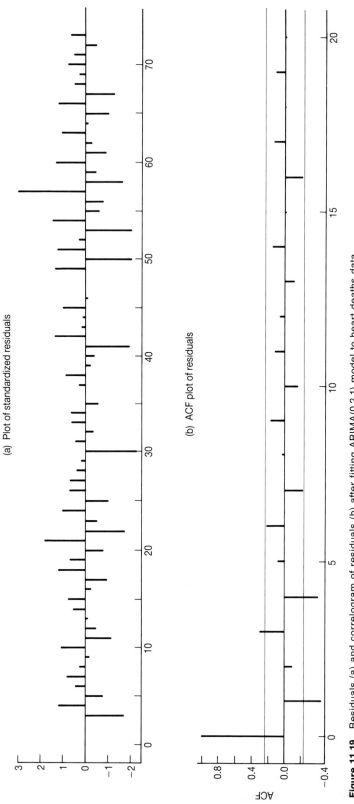

(a) Plot of standardized residuals

(b) ACF plot of residuals

Figure 11.19 Residuals (a) and correlogram of residuals (b) after fitting ARIMA(0,2,1) model to heart deaths data

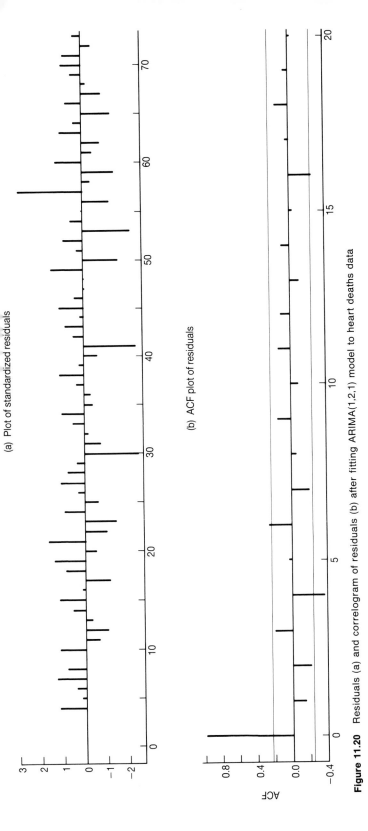

(a) Plot of standardized residuals

(b) ACF plot of residuals

Figure 11.20 Residuals (a) and correlogram of residuals (b) after fitting ARIMA(1,2,1) model to heart deaths data

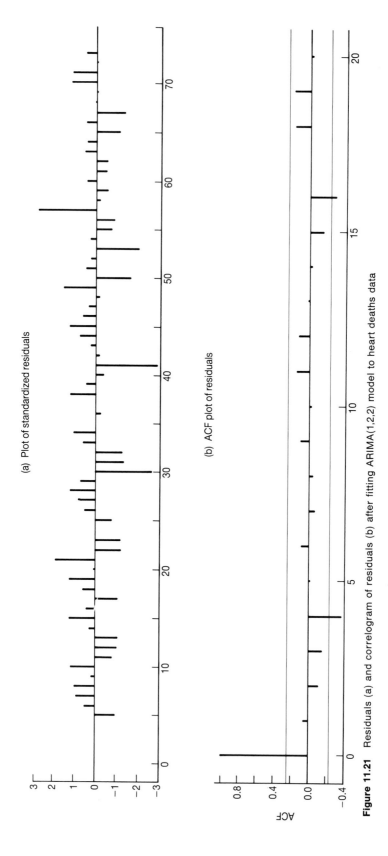

Figure 11.21 Residuals (a) and correlogram of residuals (b) after fitting ARIMA(1,2,2) model to heart deaths data

and ARIMA models. Hopefully these will serve as a useful introduction to the more comprehensive descriptions given in for example, Chatfield (1989) and Gottman (1981). Interest in time series models in medical research continues to increase and a useful review is given in Helfenstein (1991). An absorbing account of using models for forecasting is given in Tsouros and Young (1986), and a case study which uses intervention models to assess possible health effects of an environmental disaster is described in Helfenstein *et al.* (1991).

12

The Analysis of Observational Studies

12.1 Introduction

The various types of observational study used in medical investigations were introduced, and some of their associated problems discussed, in Chapter 2. In many respects the greatest difficulties with such studies are those of design and interpretation rather than analysis, and many of the methods described in previous chapters can be used with data from observational studies to answer appropriate questions. There are, however, a number of techniques which are commonly used in the analysis of observational investigations (and less frequently in the analysis of data from clinical trials, etc.), which have not been described previously. It is these methods which are covered in this chapter.

12.2 2×2 tables, relative risk and odds ratios

Evidence in medical research often comes in the form of 2×2 tables of counts. Such tables arise from the cross-classification of two dichotomous variables and are frequently used to summarize the findings of prospective, retrospective and cross-sectional studies. Table 12.1 gives an example of each.

One of the most common and important questions in observational studies involves the assessment of increased risk (if any) of incurring a particular disease if a certain factor is present. Both cohort and case-control investigations may be used to address this question and the relevant data usually forms a 2×2 table (Tables 12.1 (a) and 12.1(b) are examples). The general form for such data is shown in Table 12.2.

If the study is retrospective, the investigator begins with $a + c$ cases. A comparison group of $b + d$ controls is then selected, and the position shown in Table 12.3 is reached. Then a count of the numbers exposed and not exposed to the risk factor is determined to complete the 2×2 table. Analysis is then performed by comparing the frequency of exposure between the case and control groups (see later).

Table 12.1   2 × 2 tables from observational studies

(a) *Prospective study*

Cohort of 1000 people of whom 400 are smokers and 600 nonsmokers. Cohort observed for 20 years and 50 participants develop lung cancer of whom 45 are smokers and 5 are not.

	Lung cancer	*No lung cancer*	*Total*
Smokers	45	355	400
Nonsmokers	5	595	600
Total	50	950	1000

(b) *Retrospective study*

Adelusi (1977) describes a case-control study to investigate whether coital characteristics are associated with the subsequent development of cervical cancer. The cases were married Nigerian women with a histologic diagnosis of invasive cancer of the cervix. The control group consisted of healthy married women of a child bearing age. A questionnaire was administered to 47 cases and 173 controls, in which they were asked about their sexual habits, particularly the age at which they first had sexual intercourse.

	Cases	*Controls*	*Total*
⩽ 15 years	36	78	114
> 15 years	11	95	106
Total	47	173	220

(c) *Cross sectional study*

Senie *et al.* (1981) investigated the frequency of breast self-examination amongst women with breast cancer. The results were as follows;

Age	*Monthly*	*Frequency* *Occasionally/never*	*Total*
< 45	91	141	232
⩾ 45	259	705	984
Total	350	866	1216

Table 12.2   General form of 2 × 2 table

		Disease *Present*	*Absent*	*Total*
Risk	Present	a	b	$a + b$
factor	Absent	c	d	$c + d$
	Total	$a + c$	$b + d$	$a + b + c + d$

When the design is prospective, however, the investigator starts with the row total, $a + b$ (the exposed group) and the row total $c + d$, (the nonexposed group), and the position shown in Table 12.4 is reached. The participants are then followed forward, and eventually they fall into the disease or non-disease columns, thus again completing the table. Analysis is then performed by comparing the rate of disease occurrence (incidence) between the exposed and nonexposed groups.

Table 12.3   Initial stage in retrospective study

		Disease	
		Present(cases)	*Absent(controls)*
Risk	Present		
factor	Absent		
	Total	$a + c$	$b + d$

Table 12.4   Initial stage in prospective study

		Disease	
	Present	*Absent*	*Total*
Risk	Present (exposed)		$a + b$
factor	Absent (not-exposed)		$c + d$

After completing the 2×2 table the investigator will be most interested in estimating quantities such as the risk or probability of suffering from the disease given having been exposed to the risk factor, or the ratio of these risks for the exposed and nonexposed groups, the so called *relative risk*. In a prospective study, where a sample of the population at risk is monitored to determine the incidence of a disease, these quantities can be estimated directly from the proportion of individuals in the sample who develop the disease during the follow-up period. Consider the data in Table 12.1 (a) for example. The estimated risks of lung cancer for smokers and nonsmokers are as follows:

$$
\begin{aligned}
\text{smokers} \quad &= \quad 45/400 \quad = \quad 0.1125 \\
\text{nonsmokers} \quad &= \quad 5/600 \quad = \quad 0.0083 \\
\text{relative risk} \quad &= \quad 13.55
\end{aligned}
$$

The relevant significant test for assessing whether the incidence of lung cancer differed between smokers and nonsmokers would be the usual chi-square for a 2×2 table (see, for example, Everitt, 1992). Here, of course, the test would be highly significant. (It is important to remember that the relative risk does not measure the probability that someone with the risk factor will develop the disease. In the lung cancer and smoking data, for example, the calculated relative risk of 13.55 merely means that the probability of lung cancer is between 13 and 14 times as high for a smoker than for a nonsmoker. Smokers still have only a small chance of contracting lung cancer, however, since it is relatively uncommon.)

Now consider the 2×2 table that results from a retrospective study. Because the proportion of cases in the study will not be comparable to the proportion of diseased persons in the population, the data cannot be used to calculate risks or relative risks in the same way as described above for a prospective study. If however the disease of interest is rare, an approximation to the relative risk is given by a statistic known as the *odds ratio*, ψ, which is estimated simply as

$$\hat{\psi} = \frac{ad}{bc} \tag{12.1}$$

In Table 12.1 (b), for example, the estimate of the odds ratio is

$$\hat{\psi} = \frac{36 \times 95}{11 \times 78} = 3.99 \tag{12.2}$$

Since the odds ratio is approximately equal to the relative risk when the disease under study is rare, it is widely used as a measure of association between a disease and a risk factor, in both prospective and retrospective studies. A confidence interval for ψ can be constructed by using the estimated variance of $\ln(\hat{\psi})$, which can be shown to be

$$\mathrm{var}(\ln(\hat{\psi})) = \frac{1}{a} + \frac{1}{b} + \frac{1}{c} + \frac{1}{d} \tag{12.3}$$

By assuming normality, a 95% confidence interval for $\ln \psi$ can be constructed from

$$\ln \hat{\psi} \pm 1.96 \sqrt{\mathrm{var}(\ln \hat{\psi})} \tag{12.4}$$

Taking exponentials of the quantities in (12.4) gives the required confidence interval for ψ.

For the data in Table 12.1(b), the use of (12.3) leads to $\mathrm{var}(\ln \hat{\psi}) = 0.1420$ and to a 95% confidence interval for $\ln \psi$ of (0.6451, 2.1225). Consequently the 95% confidence interval for ψ is (1.9062, 8.3517). If age at first intercourse was *not* a risk factor for cervical cancer, the odds ratio would be one. The calculated confidence interval clearly indicates that the risk of cervical cancer in women who have first intercourse when they are relatively young, is greater by between about two and eight times, than that of women who have first intercourse when they are older than 15 years.

The interpretation of an estimated odds ratio is often made more difficult because of the possibility of obtaining a spurious association due to a lack of control of 'nuisance' or confounding variables, which are related either to the disease or to the factor under study. Consider the data on survival and amount of care received in Table 12.5. If the data are pooled over clinics, the estimated odds ratio is 2.82 with a 95% confidence interval of (1.12, 7.12). Amount of care received would appear to be a risk factor for infants' survival. For clinic A, however, the estimated odds ratio and confidence interval are 1.25 and (0.28, 5.64) respectively, and for clinic B the corresponding values are 0.99 and (0.22, 4.57). In neither clinic considered separately is there any evidence of an association between amount of care received and survival. The spurious association determined from the pooled data arises because of the relationship between amount of pre-natal care and clinic.

When a potential confounding variable is identified, a number of 2×2 tables will be available, one for each level of the variable. Within each stratum the odds ratio can be calculated as described above. To combine the individual estimates a number of approaches are possible. One is to take separate estimates of $\ln \psi$ and weight them by the reciprocal of their variance. The estimates are then combined by taking a weighted mean.

Table 12.5 Survival of infants related to amount of pre-natal care received in two clinics

		Died		Infant's survival Survived	
Amount of pre-natal care		Less	More	Less	More
Place care received	Clinic A	3	4	176	293
	Clinic B	17	2	197	23

An alternative method, and one that has several advantages (see Emerson, 1994), is due to Mantel and Haenszel (1959). This, using an obvious nomenclature, is given by

$$\hat{\psi}_{\text{pooled}} = \frac{\sum_{i=1}^{k} a_i d_i / n_i}{\sum_{i=1}^{k} b_i c_i / n_i} \qquad (12.5)$$

where k is the number of 2×2 tables involved.

Robins *et al.* (1986) proposed an estimator for the variance of $\ln(\hat{\psi}_{\text{pooled}})$ which facilitates the construction of confidence intervals. This estimator is given by

$$\text{var}(\ln(\hat{\psi}_{\text{pooled}})) = \frac{1}{2} \left[\frac{\sum_{i=1}^{k} P_i R_i}{R_+^2} + \frac{\sum_{i=1}^{k} (P_i S_i + Q_i R_i)}{R_+ S_+} + \frac{\sum_{i=1}^{k} Q_i S_i}{S_+^2} \right] \qquad (12.6)$$

where

$$
\begin{aligned}
P_i &= (a_i + d_i)/n_i, & R_+ &= \sum_{i=1}^{k} R_i, \\
Q_i &= (b_i + c_i)/n_i, & & \\
R_i &= a_i d_i / n_i, & & \\
S_i &= b_i c_i / n_i, & S_+ &= \sum_{i=1}^{k} S_i
\end{aligned}
$$

To illustrate the estimation of relative risk for stratified data, the data shown in Table 12.6 taken from Somes and O'Brian (1985), will be used. Here the interest is in the level of organic particulates in the air as a risk factor for bronchitis. The confounding variable is age which is divided into four ranges as shown. The estimates of the odds ratio for the separate age groups are as follows:

	Age			
	0–14	*15–24*	*25–39*	*40+*
$\hat{\psi}$	4.28	1.24	1.00	1.12

With these data there is clear evidence of heterogeneity in the individual estimates and, consequently, it might be inappropriate to combine them to give a pooled estimate of an assumed common odds ratio. Nevertheless, as an exercise, the pooled odds ratio and a confidence interval will be calculated using (12.5) and (12.6) above. First the Mantel–Haenszel statistic is calculated.

$$\hat{\psi}_{\text{pooled}} = \frac{19.22 + 6.85 + 3.8 + 4.16}{4.49 + 5.50 + 3.90 + 3.72} = 1.94 \qquad (12.7)$$

Table 12.6   Number of Cases of Bronchitis by level of organic particulates in the air and by age

Age	Level	Bronchitis		Total
		Yes	*No*	
0–14	High	62	915	977
	Low	7	442	449
15–24	High	20	382	402
	Low	9	214	223
25–39	High	10	172	182
	Low	7	120	127
40+	High	12	327	339
	Low	6	183	189

(Taken with permission from Somes and O'Brian, 1986)

The various terms needed for the calculation of the variance defined in (12.6) are

$$P_1 = 0.35, R_1 = 19.22, Q_1 = 0.65, S_1 = 4.49$$
$$P_2 = 0.37, R_2 = 6.85, Q_2 = 0.63, S_2 = 5.50$$
$$P_3 = 0.42, R_3 = 3.88, Q_3 = 0.58, S_3 = 3.90$$
$$P_4 = 0.37, R_4 = 4.16, Q_4 = 0.63, S_4 = 3.72$$

$$R_+ = 34.11, S_+ = 17.61$$

leading to

$$\text{var}(\ln(\hat{\psi}_{\text{pooled}})) = \frac{12.43}{2326.98} + \frac{12.43 + 10.98}{1201.35} + \frac{10.98}{620.22} = 0.0425 \tag{12.8}$$

The resulting 95% confidence interval for ψ_{pooled} is (1.30, 2.91), leading to the conclusion that the level of organic particulates in the air *is* a risk factor for bronchitis. It must be remembered however that the youngest age group is likely to be largely responsible for the pooled odds ratio being greater than one.

The method for obtaining a confidence interval for the Mantel–Haenszel statistic described above is asymptotic; its justification assumes either that the counts in the cells of the 2×2 tables are large or that the number of strata is large. Emerson (1994) describes *exact* methods for the estimation of confidence intervals based on the use of *network algorithms* as described in Mehta *et al.* (1985).

When data from a retrospective study have been collected from *matched* cases and controls the procedure for calculating the odds-ratio etc., is different from that described above. To illustrate the relevant calculations in this situation consider the data in Table 12.7 which arise from an investigation of the frequency of exposure to oral conjugated estrogens among 183 cases of endometrial cancer. Each case was matched on age, race, date of admission

Table 12.7 Frequency of exposure to
oral conjugated estrogens among 183
cases of endometrial cancer, and their
matched controls

		Controls		
		+	−	*Total*
	+	12	43	55
Cases				
	−	7	121	128
	Total	19	164	183

and hospital of admission to a suitable control not suffering from cancer. In such a matched data set the odds ratio is calculated from the *discordant pairs* only (the frequencies b and c in the general 2×2 table for such a design). The appropriate estimate is very simple being

$$\hat{\psi} = \frac{b}{c} \tag{12.9}$$

For large values of b and c an approximate confidence interval for ψ can be calculated from the $\text{var}(\ln(\hat{\psi}))$ which can be estimated from

$$\text{var}(\ln(\hat{\psi})) = \frac{1}{b} + \frac{1}{c} \tag{12.10}$$

So for the data in Table 12.6, $\hat{\psi} = 43/7 = 6.14$ with an approximate 95% confidence interval of (2.72, 13.87). (Using (12.10) to calculate the $\text{var}(\ln(\hat{\psi}))$ in this case may not be entirely appropriate because the value of c is rather small.) Miettinen (1970) shows how the odds-ratio may be calculated when there are two or more controls for each case.

When the odds ratio from either independent samples or matched samples differ across the levels of a confounding factor, that is when there is an *interaction*, it is not appropriate to combine them and the individual odds ratios for each level of the confounding variables must then be reported. If several confounding variables are identified then linear-logistic regression can be used to adjust odds ratios to take account of the confounding variables, both for prospective and retrospective studies. Details are given in Holford *et al.* (1978), Thomas (1981), Moolgavkar *et al.* (1985) and Collett (1991). Essentially the procedure for both types of investigation is as described in Chapter 5.

Logistic models can also be usefully applied to matched data when more than a single risk factor is being considered. The general form of the data in this situation is shown in Table 12.8, and the probability of disease is modelled by the linear-logistic function met in Chapter 5. Woolson and Lachenbruch (1982) show that for matched pair data, the conditional likelihood function needed as a basis for parameter estimation is determined by computing the product of n *conditional probabilities*, one for each of the n matched pairs. The required likelihood function can be shown to be the same as that for the usual logistic regression model when all values of the dichotomous dependent variable are the same, and the independent variables are the intra-pair differences on

Table 12.8 Notation for matched pair case-control data with p risk variables

Pair	Case	Control
1	$(x_{11},\ldots,x_{1p})$	$(y_{11},\ldots,y_{1p})$
2	$(x_{21},\ldots,x_{2p})$	$(y_{21},\ldots,y_{2p})$
$\vdots$	$\vdots$	$\vdots$
i	$(x_{i1},\ldots,x_{ip})$	$(y_{i1},\ldots,y_{ip})$
$\vdots$	$\vdots$	$\vdots$
n	$(x_{n1},\ldots,x_{np})$	$(y_{n1},\ldots,y_{np})$

the r risk variables. Details are given in Collett (1991). To illustrate this approach, the data in Table 12.9 will be used. These data arise from a study investigating whether known risk factors for the development of schizophrenia are more common in schizophrenics with a low age of onset, compared with an age of onset in the commonly occurring range. The risk factors considered were *complications during pregnancy and birth* (BIRTH) and *family history of psychosis* (HISTORY) both rated as simple dichotomies, present or absent. Forty people with a strict adult diagnosis of schizophrenia who had been seen for any reason by a child psychiatrist before the age of 16 were identified as the low age of onset cases. Controls, who also had schizophrenia, but who had not been seen by the psychiatric services until after the age of 21 were matched one-for-one with the cases on sex, race and socioeconomic class.

The estimated coefficients for the logistic model and their standard errors are shown in Table 12.10. It appears that only HISTORY is of importance here. The parameter estimate associated with HISTORY is the logarithm of the ratio of the odds of early onset schizophrenia occurring in a person with a family history of psychosis, relative to that for a person without such a history. So the approximate relative risk of early onset schizophrenia in a person with HISTORY = 1 relative to one with HISTORY = 0 is exp(1.547) = 4.70. The associated 95% confidence interval is (1.45, 15.2).

12.3 Log-linear models for contingency tables

The 2 × 2 table discussed in the previous section is the simplest example of a contingency table. Data arranged in the form of such tables often form a large part of many observational studies. Some examples of contingency table data are shown in Tables 12.11 and 12.12. The first of these, which has been met previously in Chapter 3, arises from cross-classifying 141 patients with brain tumours with respect to type and site of tumour. Table 12.12 results from looking at suicide deaths in terms of the method used, and the age and sex of the victim. Table 12.11 is a *two-dimensional* table involving as it does, two variables. Table 12.12 is three-dimensional.

Two-dimensional tables such as 12.11 would be assessed for the independence or otherwise of the two variables, using the familiar chi-square statistic which

Table 12.9   Case-control study risk factors
for schizophrenia

Pair	Case		Control	
	1	2	1	2
1	0	1	0	0
2	1	1	1	0
3	0	1	0	0
4	1	1	1	0
5	0	0	1	0
6	0	0	0	0
7	0	0	0	0
8	1	0	1	0
9	0	1	0	0
10	0	0	0	0
11	0	0	1	0
12	1	0	1	0
13	0	1	0	0
14	0	0	0	0
15	0	0	1	0
16	1	0	1	0
17	0	0	1	0
18	0	0	0	0
19	0	1	0	0
20	0	0	0	0
21	1	0	0	0
22	0	0	0	1
23	0	0	0	1
24	0	0	1	0
25	1	1	0	0
26	0	0	0	0
27	0	0	0	1
28	1	1	0	0
29	0	1	0	0
30	0	0	1	1
31	0	1	1	0
32	1	1	0	0
33	0	0	0	0
34	1	0	0	0
35	0	1	0	0
36	0	1	0	0
37	1	0	0	0
38	0	1	0	0
39	1	1	0	0
40	0	1	0	0

1 = Birth (1 = present, 0 = absent)
2 = History (1 = present, 0 = absent)

compares observed frequencies with those to be expected under the hypothesis of independence.

Tables with more than two dimensions generate a series of possible hypotheses — mutual independence of the variables, conditional independence of pairs of variables given the level of others, etc.; for details see Everitt (1992). Consequently the analysis of such tables is not so straightforward as that of

Table 12.10   Parameter estimates for logistic model on paired schizophrenia data

Variable	Coefficient	SE	Coef/SE	exp(coef)	LCI	UCI
BIRTH	−0.441	0.605	−0.734	0.641	0.188	2.18
HISTORY	1.547	0.579	2.67	4.70	1.45	15.2

Table 12.11   Incidence of cerebral tumours

		Type			
		A	B	C	
Site	I	23	9	6	38
	II	21	4	3	28
	III	34	24	17	75
		78	37	26	141

two-dimensional tables. Much work has been carried out in this area since the 1970s, and multidimensional contingency tables are now routinely analysed by means of *log-linear models*. These involve linear models for the log transformed counts and are, in many respects, completely analogous to the models encountered in the analysis of variance. An elementary account of such models is given in Everitt (1992) and a more complete account in Fienberg (1981). Here attention is restricted to a brief description of the various log-linear models that might be applied to a three-demensional table in which the expected values of the frequencies are $F_{ijk}, i = 1, 2, \ldots, r; j = 1, 2, \ldots, c; k = 1, 2, \ldots, l$ Consider first the so called *saturated* model for such a table

$$\ln F_{ijk} = u + u_{1(i)} + u_{2(j)} + u_{3(k)} + u_{12(ij)} + u_{13(ik)} + u_{23(jk)} + u_{123(ijk)} \quad (12.11)$$

The parameters in this model represent main effects of each variable (u_1, u_2, u_3),

Table 12.12   Suicide behaviour. Age by sex by cause of death

Age group	*Causes of death*					
	(1) Solid or liquid matter	(2) Gas	(3) Hanging, strangling, suffocating, drowning	(4) Gun, knives, explosives	(5) Jumping	(6) Other
Male						
10–39 (A1)	398	121	455	155	55	124
40–70 (A2)	399	82	797	168	51	82
> 70 (A3)	93	6	316	33	26	14
Female						
10–39 (A1)	259	15	95	14	40	38
40–70 (A2)	450	13	450	26	71	60
> 70 (A3)	154	5	185	7	38	10

first-order interaction effects (u_{12}, u_{13}, u_{23}) and second-order interaction effects (u_{123}). The nomenclature used for the parameters is that the numerical subscripts represent variables, and the alphabetic subscripts, categories of these variables. When the latter are omitted, all categories are implied. Fitting the saturated model in (12.12) to a three-dimensional table would result in a set of estimated expected values, identical to the observed values, leading to a zero value for the chi-square statistic and a perfect fit of the model to the data. Hence the term saturated model. If no simpler model (that is one with some of the parameters in (12.12) equal to zero), provided an adequate fit to the data, it would imply that the association between each pair of variables differed in degree and/or direction in levels of the remaining variable.

In general a series of models will be fitted to a table in a search for the one that is most parsimonious, in the sense of providing an acceptable fit with the fewest number of parameters. The hypothesis of no second order interaction, for example, would be

$$H_0 : u_{123} = 0 \qquad (12.12)$$

which implies that the model

$$\ln F_{ijk} = u + u_{1(i)} + u_{2(j)} + u_{3(k)} + u_{12(ij)} + u_{13(ik)} + u_{23(jk)} \qquad (12.13)$$

adequately describes the data. Estimated expected frequencies under the model may be found by maximum likelihood methods using the *iterative proportional fitting* (IPF) algorithm (see Everitt, 1992, for details). If such a model is chosen for the data, it implies that each pair of variables is associated, and that these associations are of the same strength and direction in each level of the remaining variable.

The simplest model of interest is that corresponding to the hypothesis that the three variables are mutually independent, namely

$$\ln F_{ijk} = u + u_{1(i)} + u_{2(j)} + u_{3(k)} \qquad (12.14)$$

In this case maximum likelihood estimates of the expected frequencies may be found explicitly from various marginal totals in the observed table (see Everitt, 1992, for details). The same estimates will also be given by the IPF algorithm in a single iteration, however.

Each model of interest can be assessed by comparing the estimated expected frequencies and the corresponding observed values by means of Pearson's chi-square statistic or an alternative, *likelihood ratio*, goodness-of-fit measure. (Again see Everitt, 1992, for details). Since the number of possible models increases rapidly with the number of dimensions of a multidimensional table, procedures for choosing between competing models become of considerable importance when fitting log-linear models to a contingency table. Perhaps the simplest approach is to assess the effect of adding extra parameters to the model currently under consideration, by examining the difference in the likelihood ratio measure of fit for the two models, and testing the significance of the difference. The model with more parameters would only be preferred if it provided a significantly improved fit over the simpler model. More complex procedures for choosing a particular model are described in Aitkin (1978). Estimates of the parameters in log-linear models are obtained in a similar fashion to estimates of the parameters in analysis of variance models and

Table 12.13   Expected values for mutual independence model

Sex	Age	Method						
		solid	*gas*	*hang*	*gun*	*jump*	*other*	*Total*
males	a1	371.9	51.3	487.5	85.5	59.6	69.6	1125.4
	a2	556.9	76.9	730.0	128.0	89.3	104.2	1685.3
	a3	186.5	25.7	244.4	42.9	29.9	34.9	564.3
Total	—	1115.2	154.0	1462.0	256.4	178.8	208.7	3375.0
females	a1	212.7	29.4	278.8	48.9	34.1	39.8	643.6
	a2	318.5	44.0	417.5	73.2	51.0	59.6	963.7
	a3	106.6	14.7	139.8	24.5	17.1	20.0	322.7
Total	—	637.8	88.0	836.0	146.6	102.2	119.3	1930.0

generally involve combinations of the means of the log linear transformed estimated expected values. (For further details see Everitt, 1992).

To illustrate the fitting of log-linear models, the data in Table 12.12 will be used. The first model considered is that in which the three variables, age, sex and method of suicide are independent of one another, that is the model specified in (12.15). The estimated expected values under this model are shown in Table 12.13. The goodness-of-fit measure indicates the very poor fit of this model-Pearson chi-square $= 747.37$, d.f. $= 27$, $p < 0.001$: likelihood ratio chi-square $= 790.30$, d.f. $= 27$, $p < 0.001$. Models of increasing complexity now need to be considered. In general only *hierarchical models* are of interest, these being such that whenever a higher-order effect is included in the model the lower-order effects comprised from variables in the higher-order effect are also included. So, for example, if a term u_{123} is included in a model, terms $u_{12}, u_{13}, u_{23}, u_1, u_2$ and u_3 must also be included. This restriction to hierarchical models arises essentially from the constraints imposed by the maximum likelihood estimation procedures, details of which are given in Bishop *et al.* (1975).

The results of fitting all possible hierarchical models from mutual independence to the presence of a second order interaction are shown in Table 12.14. In this table the log-linear models are identified by showing the most complex term in the model. Comparing the saturated model with the u_{12}, u_{13}, u_{23} model shows that allowing a second-order interaction decreases the goodness-of-fit criterion by 14.90 with a decrease in degrees of freedom of 10. This decrease is not significant, and so it appears that no second-order interaction term is needed. Comparing the measure of fit of the u_{12}, u_{13}, u_{23} model with the remaining simpler models, however, it is clear that none of the simpler models provide an adequate fit. For these data the model specified in (12.13) is selected as most satisfactory. The model implies that each pair of variables is associated, but the degree and direction of the association is the same in each level of the remaining variable. Estimated expected values under this model are shown in Table 12.15.

As with other model fitting procedures described in earlier chapters, simply assessing whether or not a model fits by examination of a single goodness-of-fit

Table 12.14 Results from fitting all hierarchical log-linear models to suicide data

Model	d.f.	LR chi-square	p	Pearson chi-square	p
u_1, u_2, u_3	27	790.30	< 0.001	747.37	< 0.001
u_1, u_{23}	25	658.89	< 0.001	635.96	< 0.001
u_2, u_{13}	22	424.59	< 0.001	396.60	< 0.001
u_3, u_{12}	17	520.41	< 0.001	485.33	< 0.001
u_{12}, u_{13}	12	154.70	< 0.001	151.23	< 0.001
u_{13}, u_{23}	20	293.18	< 0.001	278.55	< 0.001
u_{23}, u_{12}	15	389.00	< 0.001	369.54	< 0.001
u_{12}, u_{13}, u_{23}	10	14.90	0.1357	15.40	0.1182

Variable 1 is METHOD, variable 2 is AGEGROUP and variable 3 is SEX.

Table 12.15 Expected values for the u_{12}, u_{13}, u_{23} model

Sex	Age	Method						
		solid	gas	hang	gun	jump	other	Total
males	a1	410.9	122.7	439.2	156.4	56.8	122.0	1308.0
	a2	379.4	77.6	819.9	163.3	51.1	84.7	1579.0
	a3	99.7	8.7	308.9	33.4	24.1	13.3	488.0
Total	—	890.0	209.0	1568.0	356.0	132.0	220.0	3375.0
females	a1	246.1	13.3	110.8	12.6	38.2	40.0	461.0
	a2	469.6	17.4	427.1	27.7	70.9	57.3	1070.0
	a3	147.3	2.3	192.1	6.6	39.9	10.7	399.0
Total	—	863.0	33.0	730.0	47.0	149.0	108.0	1930.0

statistic is usually not adequate. As always the examination of residuals is important. For log-linear models there are a number of ways of calculating informative residuals. Perhaps the most useful are the *standardized deviates* defined as

$$(O - E)/\sqrt{E} \tag{12.15}$$

where O represents an observed value and E the corresponding estimated expected value under a particular model. Such residuals have an approximately standard normal distribution and so values outside the range -2.0 to 2.0 suggest cells where the current model is inadequate. Tables 12.16 and 12.17 show the standardized deviates for the mutual independence model, u_1, u_2, u_3, and the model chosen for the data, u_{12}, u_{13}, u_{23}. In the first of these tables there are many values outside the $-2, 2$ range. In Table 12.17, no values fall outside these limits, confirming that this model fits the data very well.

Table 12.16 Standardized residuals for mutual independence model

Sex	Age	Method					
		solid	*gas*	*hang*	*gun*	*jump*	*other*
males	a1	1.4	9.7	−1.5	7.5	−0.6	6.5
	a2	−6.7	0.6	2.5	3.5	−4.1	−2.2
	a3	−6.8	−3.9	4.6	−1.5	−0.7	−3.5
females	a1	3.2	−2.6	−11.0	−5.0	1.0	−0.3
	a2	7.4	−4.7	1.6	−5.5	2.8	0.1
	a3	4.6	−2.5	3.8	−3.5	5.1	−2.2

Table 12.17 Standardized residuals for the u_{12}, u_{13}, u_{23} model

Sex	Age	Method					
		solid	*gas*	*hang*	*gun*	*jump*	*other*
males	a1	−0.6	−0.2	0.8	−0.1	−0.2	0.2
	a2	1.0	0.5	−0.8	0.1	−0.0	−0.3
	a3	−0.7	−0.9	0.4	−0.1	0.4	0.2
females	a1	0.8	0.5	−1.5	0.4	0.3	−0.3
	a2	−0.9	−1.1	1.1	−0.3	0.0	0.4
	a3	0.6	1.8	−0.5	0.1	−0.3	−0.2

12.4 Summary

Many of the problems of observational studies involve design and interpretation rather than analysis. There are, however, a number of techiques particularly relevant to such studies and several of these have been briefly discussed in this chapter. More detailed accounts of the analysis of observational studies are given in Fleiss (1986).

Appendix

Statistical Software

Most of the methods of analysis described in this book could not be applied routinely without the aid of a computer and some relevant software. Fortunately, many excellent statistical packages are available which allow investigators access to an enormous variety of statistical methods. (Unfortunately such general availability does not necessarily imply that the correct or relevant or indeed sensible, analysis will be carried out!) Some packages are very general, for example, the 'big three', BMDP, SPSS and SAS. Others are designed more for a specific problem or type of data (for example, STATXACT). Some packages are extremely easy to use (particularly those that are 'menu driven'), others require more application but can generally offer more 'focused' analyses. Reviews of statistical software now appear regularly in statistical journals, and it is not intended that this Appendix try to duplicate this material. A partial least of available packages and a brief description of their facilities may be helpful, however, and this is what is included here.

General statistical packages

(a) BMDP

BMDP (Biomedical Package) consists of a series of programs, each designed for a particular type of statistical analysis, for example: multiple regression, logistic regression, analysis of repeated measures, survival analysis, factor analysis, discriminant function analysis and log-linear models. The manuals describing the package are generally excellent, and the package is reviewed in Lovie (1988) and Everitt (1991). Relevant addresses are:

BMDP Statistical Software Inc.,
1440 Sepulveda Boulevard,
Suite 316,
Los Angeles, CA 90025, USA

BMDP Statistical Software,
Cork Technology Park,
Model Farm Road,
Cork, Ireland

(b) SAS

SAS (Statistical Analysis System) is a computer software system for data processing and data analysis. The package has particularly extensive facilities for file handling as well as allowing for most types of statistical analysis including regression, analysis of variance, survival analysis, time series analysis, etc. A detailed review of the package is given in Lovie (1989) and information about the package is available from:

SAS Institute Inc.,
Sales and Marketing Division,
SAS Campus Drive,
Cary, NC 27513, USA

SAS Software Ltd.,
Wittington House,
Henley Road,
Marlow,
Buckinghamshire, SL7 2EB, UK

(c) SPSS

SPSS (Statistical Package for Social Scientists) is again a comprehensive data analysis system. The scope of the package is broadly similar to that of BMDP and SAS, and the package can be used to apply regression, analysis of variance, multivariate analysis, correspondence analysis, etc. A review of the SPSS package is given by Lovie (1988). Details of the package can be obtained from:

SPSS, Inc.,
444 N Michigan Avenue,
Chicago, IL 60611, USA

SPSS UK Ltd.,
SPSS House,
5 London Street,
Chertsey,
Surrey, KT16 8AP, UK

(d) MINITAB

MINITAB is a general-purpose statistical computing system developed to make it easier to use computers for the analyses of data. Its range of methods is not as extensive as those in BMDP, SAS or SPSS, but do include multiple regression, analysis of variance and time series analysis. The ease of use of the package makes it an excellent choice for teaching. MINITAB is reviewed in Lovie (1992). Information about the package is available from:

MINITAB Statistical Software,
3081 Enterprise Drive,
State College,
PA 16801, USA

(e) STATGRAPHICS

STATGRAPHICS allows the application of analysis of variance, regression analysis, time series analysis and many other statistical methods. Its graphical facilities are particularly extensive. Details are available from:

STSC Inc.,
2115 East Jefferson St.,
Nickville, MD 20852, USA

(f) SYSTAT

SYSTAT is a further comprehensive package of statistical techniques including cluster analysis, principal components analysis and regression. The graphical facilities in the package are extensive and powerful. The documentation is excellent. A review of the software is given in Lovie (1991a). Details of the software can be obtained from:

SYSTAT,
1800 Sterman Avenue,
Evanston, IL 60201-3793, USA

Specialized software

(a) STATXACT

STATXACT is a statistical package for exact nonparametric inference. The most important feature of STATXACT distinguishing it from most other statistical software is that it computes *exact p values* for a number of frequently used hypothesis testing procedures for comparing two or more populations. STATXACT is particularly useful when data are sparse. The accompanying user manual contains numerous examples and clear guidelines on when each test is applicable. The package is reviewed in Marsh (1991). Further details are available from:

Cyrus R. Mehta,
Cytel Software Corporation,
137 Erie St.,
Cambridge, MA 02139, USA

(b) EGRET

EGRET is a package particularly suitable for the analysis of data from epidemiological studies. The package provides logistic regression, Cox's regression, Kaplan–Meier estimation of survival curves, etc. A brochure about the software is available from:

Statistics and Epidemiology Research Corporation,
909 Northeast 43rd Street,
Suite 202,
Seattle, WA 98105, USA.

(c) GLIM

GLIM (Generalized Linear Interactive Modelling) was written to enable the family of generalized linear models described by Nelder and Wedderburn (1972) to be fitted to data. This general model includes multiple regression and logistic regression as special cases. Macros can be created to enable complex non-standard methods of analysis to be applied. GLIM is a first rate package particularly for applied statisticians. Details of the latest version of the software are available from:

NAG Ltd.,
Wilkinson House,
Jordan Hill Road,
Oxford, OX2 8DR, UK

NAG Inc.,
1400 Opus Place,
Suite 200,
Downers Grave
IL 60515-5702, USA

Statistical languages

(a) GENSTAT

GENSTAT (General Statistical Program) includes many statistical methods such as analysis of variance, regression and time series analysis but also provides a powerful programming environment for creating more tailored methods of data analysis, and for implementing methods not available in general statistical packages. Details are available from the same address as given for GLIM.

(b) S-PLUS

S-PLUS is a commercially enhanced and supported release of the Bell Laboratories' S statistical package. S-PLUS is both a statistical package — that is a collection of data analysis tools — and a powerful programming language for creating new tools. The package is very strong on exploratory data analysis procedures and graphics. Recent additions have also made the statistical modelling component of the package excellent. S-PLUS is reviewed in Lovie (1991b) and Therneau (1990). Addresses for details are:

Statsci Europe,
52 Sandfield Road,
Headington,
Oxford, OX3 7RJ, UK.

Statistical Sciences Inc.,
PO Box 85625,
Seattle, WA 98145-1625, USA

References

Adelusi, B. (1977). Carcinoma of the cervix uteri in Ibadan: coital characteristics. *International Journal of Gynaecology and Obstetrics*, **15**, 5–11.

Aitkin, M. (1978). The analysis of unbalanced cross-classifications, *Journal of the Royal Statistical Society, Series A*, **141**, 195–223.

Alderson, M. (1983). *An Introduction to Epidemiology*, Second Edition, Macmillan London.

Allen, D.M. (1971). Mean square error of prediction as a criterion for selecting variables. *Technometrics*, **13**, 469–75.

Allen, G.M. (1983). Clinical diagnosis of the acute stroke syndrome. *Quarterly Journal of Medicine*, **52**, 515–23.

Allison, P.D. (1984). *Event History Analysis Regression for Longitudinal Event Data*, Sage Publications, London.

Altman, D.G. (1980a). Statistics and ethics in medical research I: Misuse of statistics is unethical. *British Medical Journal*, **281**, 1181–4.

Altman, D.G. (1980b) Statistics and ethics in medical research: III. How large a sample? *British Medical Journal*, **281**, 1336–8.

Altman, D.G. (1982). Statistics in medical journals. *Statistics in Medicine*, **1**, 59–71.

Altman, D.G. (1991). *Practical Statistics for Medical Research*, Chapman and Hall, London.

Ambroz, A., Chalmers, T.C., Smith, H., Schroeder, B., Freiman, J.A. and Shareck, E.P. (1978). Deficiencies of randomized clinical trials. *Clinical Research*, **26**, 280A.

Anderberg, M.R. (1973). *Cluster Analysis for Applications*, Academic Press, New York.

Andersen, B. (1990). *Methodological Errors in Medical Research*. Blackwell Scientific Publications, Oxford.

Anderson, J.A. (1972) Separate sample logistic discrimination. *Biometrika*, **59**, 19–35.

Anderson, N.H. (1963) Comparison of different populations: resistance to extinction and transfer. *Psychological Review*, **70**, 162–79.

Armitage, P. and Berry, G. (1987). *Statistical Methods in Medical Research*, Blackwell, Oxford.

Armitage, P. and Hills, M. (1982). The two-period crossover trial. *The Statistician*, **31**, 119–31.

Armitage, P., McPherson, C.K. and Copas, J.C. (1969). Statistical studies of prognosis in advanced breast cancer. *Journal Chronic Disorders*, **22**, 343–60.

Atkinson, A.C. (1987). *Plots, Transformations and Regression*, Oxford Science Publications, Oxford.

Balarajan, R., Yuen, P. and Bewley, B.R. (1985). Smoking and state of health, *British Medical Journal*, **291**, 1682.

Barer, D.H., Cruckshank, J.M., Ebrahim, S.B. and Mitchell, J.R. (1988). Low dose beta blockade in acute stroke (BEST trial): an evaluation, *British Medical Journal*, **296**, 737–41.

Baum, M.L., Arush, D.S., Chalmers, T.C., Sacks, H.S., Smith, H. and Fagerström, R.M. (1981). A survey of clinical trials of antibiotic prophylaxis in colon surgery: evidence against further use of no-treatment controls. *New England Journal of Medicine*, **305**, 795–99.

Begg, C.B. and Berlin, J.A. (1988). Publication bias a problem in interpreting medical data. *Journal of the Royal Statistical Society Series A.*, **151**, 419–63.

Bellingham, K. and Gillies, P. (1993). Evaluation of an AIDS education programme for young adults, *Journal of Epidermiology and Community Health*, **47**, 134–8.

Bentley, J.M., Cormier, P. and Oler, J. (1983). The rural dental health program: the effect of a school-based, dental health education program on children's utilization of dental services. *American Journal of Public Health*, **73**, 500–5.

Bhargava, S.K., Ramji, S., Kumar, A., Mohan, M. and Marwah, J. (1985). Mid-arm and chest circumferences at birth as predictors of low birth weight and neonatal mortality in the community. *British Medical Journal*, **291**, 1617–19.

Bishop, S.H. and Jones, B. (1984). A review of higher order crossover designs. *Journal of Applied Statistics*, **11**, 29–50.

Bishop, Y.M.M., Fienberg, S.E. and Holland, F.W. (1975). *Discrete Multivariate Analysis*. Institute of Technology Press, Massachusetts.

Bosaeus, E., Matousek, M. and Petersen, I. (1977). Correlation between paedopsychiatric findings and EEG-variables in well-functioning children of ages 5 to 16 years. An EEG frequency analysis study. *Scandanavian Journal of Psychology*, **18**, 140–7.

Box, G.E.P. (1950). Problems in the analysis of growth and wear curves. *Biometrics*, **6**, 326–89.

Box, G.E.P. and Jenkins, G.M. (1970). *Time Series Analysis: Forecasting and Control*, Holden-Day, San Francisco.

Box, G.E.P. and Tiao, G.C. (1975). Intervention analysis with applications to economic and environmental problems. *Journal of the American Statistical Association*, **70**, 70–9.

Bracken, M.B. (1987). Clinical trials and the acceptance of uncertainty, *British Medical Journal*, **294**, 1111–12.

Bradford Hill, A. (1962). *Statistical Methods in Clinical and Preventive Medicine*, Livingstone, Edinburgh.

Bradford Hill – see also under Hill.

Brazier, M.A. (1956). Electroencephalography. *Progression in Neuro Psychiatry*, N.Y., **10**, 279–92.

Breddin, K., Loew, D., Lechner, K. and Uberla, E.W. (1979). Secondary prevention of myocardial infarction. Comparison of acetylsalicylic acid, Phenprocoumon and placebo. A multicenter two-year prospective study. *Thrombosis and Haemostasis*, **41**, 225–36.

Brooke, O.G., Anderson, H.R., Bland, M.J., Peacock, J.L. and Stewart, C.M. (1989). Effects on birthweight of smoking, alcohol, caffeine, socioeconomic factors and psychosocial stress, *British Medical Journal*, **298**, 795.

Brown, B.W. (1980). The crossover experiment for clinical trials. *Biometrics*, **36**, 69–79.

Burkhardt, R. and Kienle, G. (1978). Controlled clinical trials and medical ethics, *Lancet*, **(ii)**, 1356–9.

Cassagrande, J.T., Pike, M.C. and Smith, P.G. (1978). The power function of the 'exact' test for comparing two binominal proportions. *Applied Statistics*, **27**, 176–80.

Chalmers, T.C. and Lau, J. (1993). Meta-analytic stimulus for changes in clinical trials. *Statistical Methods in Medical Research*, **2**, 161–72.

Chalmers, T.C., Berrier, J., Sacks, H.S., Levin, H., Reitman, D. and Nagalingham, R. (1987). Meta analysis of clinical trials as a scientific discipline II: Replicate variability and comparison of studies that agree and disagree. *Statistics in Medicine*, **6**, 733–44.

Chalmers, T.C., Matta, R.J., Smith, H. and Kunzer, A. (1977). Evidence favouring the use of anticoagulants in the hospital phase of acute myocardial infarction. *New England Journal of Medicine*, **297**, 1091–96.

Chatfield, C. (1989). *The Analysis of Time Series*, 4th Edition, Chapman and Hall, London.

Chatterjee, S. and Price, B. (1991). *Regression Analysis by Example*, 2nd Edn, Wiley, New York.

Chi, P.Y., Bristol, D.R. and Castellona, J.V. (1986). A clinical trial with an interim analysis. *Statistics in Medicine*, **5**, 387–92.

Clayton, D. and Hills, M. (1987). A two-period crossover trial. In *The Statistical Consultant in Action*, D.J. Hand and B.S. Everitt, (eds). Cambridge University Press, Cambridge.

Cochran, W.G. and Cox, G.M. (1966). *Experimental Designs* (3rd edn), Wiley, New York.

Cohen, J. (1960). A coefficient of agreement for nominal scales. *Educational and Psychological Measurement*, **20**, 37–46.

Cohen, J. (1977). *Statistical Power Analysis for the Behavioural Sciences*. Academic Press, New York.

Collett, D. (1991). *Modelling Binary Data*, Chapman and Hall, London.

Colton, T. (1974). *Statistics in Medicine*, Little, Brown and Company, Boston.

Connett, J.E., Smith, J.A. and McHugh, R.B. (1987). Sample size and power for pair matched case-control studies. *Statistics in Medicine*, **6**, 53–9.

Cook, D.G. and Pocock, S.J. (1987). Consultancy in a medical school illustrated by a clinical trial for treatment of primary biliary cirrhosis. In *The Statistical Consultant in Action*, D.J. Hand and B.S. Everitt (eds). Cambridge University Press, Cambridge.

Cook, R.D. and Weisberg, S. (1982). *Residuals and Influence in Regression,* Chapman and Hall, London.

Cormack, R.M. (1971). A review of classification. *Journal of the Royal Statistical Society, Series A,* **134,** 321–67.

Coste, J., Spira, A., Duametiere, P. and Paolaggi, J.B. (1991). Clinical and psychological diversity of non-specific low-back pain. A new approach towards the classification of clinical subgroups. *Journal of Clinical Epidemiology,* **44,** 1233–45.

Cox, D.R. (1959). The analysis of exponentially distributed life times with two types of failure. *Journal of the Royal Statistical Society, Series B,* **21,** 411–21.

Cox, D.R. (1972). Regression models and life tables. *Journal of the Royal Statistical Society B,* **34,** 187–220.

Cox, D.R. and Oakes, D. (1984). *Analysis of Survival Data,* Chapman and Hall, London.

Cox, D.R. and Snell, E.J. (1989). *Analysis of Binary Data,* Second edition, Chapman and Hall, London.

Crichton, N.J. and Hinde, J.P. (1989). Correspondence analysis as a screening method for indicants for clinical diagnosis, *Statistics in Medicine,* **8,** 1351–62.

Crowley, J. and Hu, M. (1977). Covariance analysis of heart transplant survival data. *Journal of the American Statistical Association,* **72,** 27–36.

Day, N.E. (1969). Estimating the components of a mixture of normal distributions, *Biometrika,* **56,** 463–74.

Day, N.E. and Kerridge, D.R. (1967). A general maximum likelihood discriminant. *Biometrics,* **23,** 313–23.

Dennerstein, L., Spencer-Gardner, C., Gotts, G., Brown, J.B. and Smith, M.A. (1985). Progesterone and the premenstrual syndrome: a double blind cross-over trial. *British Medical Journal,* **290,** 1617–21.

Donner, A. (1984). Approaches to sample size estimations in the design of clinical trials — a review. *Statistics in Medicine,* **3,** 199–214.

Donner, A. and Eliasziw, M. (1987). Sample size requirements for reliability studies. *Statistics in Medicine,* **6,** 441–8.

Draper, N. and Smith, H. (1981). *Applied Regression Analysis,* Wiley, New York.

Dumermuth, G., Gasser, A., Hecker, A., Herdan, M. and Lange, B. (1976). Exploration of EEG components in the beta frequency range. In P. Kellaway and I. Petersen etc. *Quantitative Analytic Studies in Epilepsy.* Raven Press, New York.

Dunn, G. (1986). Patterns of psychiatric diagnosis in general practice: the second national morbidity survey. *Psychological Medicine,* **16,** 573–81.

Dunn, G. (1989). *Design and Analysis of Reliability Studies: Statistical Evaluation of Measurement Errors,* Edward Arnold, Sevenoaks.

Dunn, G., Everitt, B.S. and Pickles, A. (1993). *Modelling Covariances and Latent Variables Using EQS.* Chapman and Hall, London.

Dunstan, F.D.J. (1993). Time Series Analysis, In *Biological Data Analysis: a Practical Approach,* J.C. Fry (ed), Oxford University Press, Oxford.

Edelbrook, C. (1979). Comparing the accuracy of hierarchical clustering algorithms: The problem of classifying everybody. *Multivariate Behavioural*

Research, **14**, 367–84.

Ekström, D., Quade, D. and Golden, R.N. (1990). Statistical analysis of repeated measures in psychiatric research, *Archives of General Psychiatry*, **47**, 770–2.

Eliasziw, M. and Donner, A. (1987). A cost-function approach to the design of reliability studies. *Statistics in Medicine*, **6**, 647–56.

Emerson, J.D. (1994). Combining estimates of the odds ratio: the state of the art. *Statistical Methods in Medical Research*. In press.

Everitt, B.S. (1968). Moments of the statistics kappa and weighted kappa. *British Journal of Mathematical and Statistical Psychology*, **21**, 97–103.

Everitt, B.S. (1977). *The Analysis of Contingency Tables*. Chapman and Hall, London.

Everitt, B.S. (1979). Cluster analysis: A discussion of some unresolved problems and possible future developments. *Biometrics*, **35**, 169–81.

Everitt, B.S. (1991). BMDP PC-90 Software Review, *Statistics and Computing*, **1**, 71–73.

Everitt, B.S. (1992) *The Analysis of Contingency Tables*, 2nd Edition, Chapman and Hall, London.

Everitt, B.S. (1993) *Cluster Analysis*, 3rd edition, Edward Arnold, Sevenoaks.

Everitt B.S. and Dunn, G. (1991). *Applied Multivariate Data Analysis*, Edward Arnold, Sevenoaks, England.

Everitt B.S. and Hand, D.J. (1981). *Finite Mixture Distributions*, Chapman and Hall, London.

Everitt B.S., Gourlay, A.J. and Kendell, R.E. (1971). An attempt at validation of traditional psychiatric syndromes by cluster analysis. *British Journal of Psychiatry*, **119**, 399–412.

Falissard, B. and Lellouch, J. (1991). Some extensions to a new approach for interim analysis in clinical trials. *Statistics in Medicine*, **10**, 949–57.

Farewell, V.T. (1985). Some remarks on the analysis of crossover trials with a binary response. *Applied Statistics*, **34**, 121–8.

Feldman, S., Klein, D.F. and Honigfeld, G. (1972). The reliability of a decision tree technique applied to psychiatric diagnosis. *Biometrics*, **28**, 831–40.

Fenwick, P.B.C., Michie, P., Dollimore, J. and Fenton, G.W. (1971). Mathematical simulation of the electroencephalogram using an autoregressive series. *Bio-Medical Computing*, **2**, 281–307.

Fidler, V. (1984). Changeover clinical trial with binary data: mixed-model based comparison tests. *Biometrics*, **40**, 1063–70.

Fienberg, S.E. (1981). *The Analysis of Cross-Classified Categorical Data* (2nd edn), MIT Press, Cambridge, Massachusetts.

Finn, J.D. (1974). *A General Model for Multivariate Analysis*, Holt, Rinehart and Winston, New York.

Finney, D.J. (1990). Repeated measurements: what is measured and what repeats? *Statistics in Medicine*, **9**, 639–44.

Fisher, L.D. and van Belle, G. (1993). *Biostatistics: Methodology for the Health Sciences*. John Wiley, New York.

Fisher, R.A. (1932). *Statistical Methods for Research Workers* (4th edn), Oliver and Boyd, Edinburgh.

Fisher, R.A. (1936). The use of multiple measurements in taxonomic problems. *Annals of Eugenics*, **7**, 179–88.

Fleiss, J.L. (1965). Estimating the accuracy of dichotomous judgements. *Psychometrika*, **30**, 469–79.

Fleiss, J.L. (1973). *Statistical Methods for Rates and Proportions*, Wiley, New York.

Fleiss, J.L. (1975). Measuring agreement between judges on the presence or absence of a trait. *Biometrics*, **31**, 651–9.

Fleiss, J.L. (1986). *The Design and Analysis of Clinical Experiments*, Wiley, New York.

Fleiss, J.L. (1987). Discussion contribution to Light, R.J. *Statistics in Medicine*, **6**, 221–28.

Fleiss, J.L. (1993). The statistical basis of meta-analysis. *Statistical Methods in Medical Research*, **2**, 121–45.

Fleiss, J.L. and Cuzick, J. (1979). The reliability of dichotomous judgements: unequal numbers of judgements per subject. *Applied Psychological Measurement*, **3**, 537–42.

Fleiss, J.L. and Tanur, J.M. (1972). The analysis of covariance in psychopathology. In M. Hammer, K. Salzinger and S. Sutton (eds), *Psychopathology*, Wiley, New York.

Fleiss, J.L., Cohen, J. and Everitt, B.S. (1969). Large sample standard errors of kappa and weighted kappa. *Psychological Bulletin*, **72**, 323–7.

Freeman, C.P.L., Barry, F., Dunkfeld-Turnbull, J. and Henderson, A. (1988). Controlled trial of psychotherapy for bulimia nervosa, *British Medical Journal*, **296**, 521–5.

Freiman, J.A., Chalmers, T.C. and Smith, H. (1978). The importance of beta, the type II error and sample size in the design and interpretation of the randomized control trial: survey of 'negative' trials. *New England Journal of Medicine*, **299**, 690–4.

Frison, L. and Pocock, S.J. (1992). Repeated measures in clinical trials: analysis using mean summary statistics and its implication for design. *Statistics in Medicine*, **11**, 1685–704.

Gardner, M.J. and Altman, D.G. (1986). Confidence intervals rather than *P* values: estimation rather than hypothesis testing. *British Medical Journal*, **292**, 746–50.

Gart, J.J. (1969). An exact test for comparing matched proportions in crossover designs. *Biometrika*, **56**, 75–80.

Gehan, E.A. (1965). A generalized Wilcoxon tests for comparing arbitrarily singly censored samples. *Biometrika*, **52**, 203–23.

Gehan, E.A. (1983). The evaluation of therapies: historical control studies. *Statistics in Medicine*, **4**, 315–24.

Gehan, E.A. and Freireich, E.J. (1974). Non-randomized controls in cancer clinical trials. *New England Journal of Medicine*, **290**, 198–203.

Gerbarg, Z.B. and Horiwitz, R.I. (1988). Resolving conflicting clinical trials: guidelines for meta analysis. *Journal of Clinical Epidemiology*, **41**, 502–9.

Gilbert, E.S. (1968). On discrimination using qualitative variables. *Journal of the American Statistical Association*, **63**, 1399–412.

Golding, J. Paterson, M. and Kinlen, L.J. (1990). Factors associated with childhood cancer in a national cohort study, *British Journal of Cancer*, **62**, 304–08.

Goldman, L., Weinburg, M., Weisberg, M., Olshen, R., Cook, E.F., Sargent,

R.K., Medical House Staffs at Yale-New Haven and Brigham Women's Hospital (1982). A computer derived protocol to aid in the diagnosis of emergency room patients with chest pain. *New England Journal of Medicine*, **307**, 588–96.

Goodman, L.A. (1974) Exploratory latent structure analysis using both identifiable and unidentifiable models. *Biometrika*, **61**, 215–31.

Gornbein, J.A., Lazaro, C.G. and Little, R.J.A. (1992). Incomplete data in repeated measures analysis. *Statistical Methods in Medical Research*, **1**, 275–95.

Gottman, J.M. (1981). *Time Series Analysis: a comprehensive introduction for social scientists*, Cambridge University Press.

Gower, J.C. (1985). Measures of similarity, dissimilarity and distance. In *Encyclopedia of Statistical Sciences*, Volume 5, S. Kotz, N.L. Johnston and C.B. Read (eds). John Wiley, New York.

Green, P.J. (1984). Iteratively reweighted least squares for maximum likelihood estimation and some robust and resistant alternatives (with discussion). *Journal of the Royal Statistical Society, Series B*, **46**, 149–92.

Greenacre, M.J. (1984). *Theory and Application of Correspondence Analysis*, Academic Press, London.

Greenacre, M.J. (1992). Correspondence analysis in medical research. *Statistical Methods in Medical Research*, **1**, 97–117.

Greenhouse, S.W. and Geisser, S. (1959). On methods in the analysis of profile data. *Psychometrika*, **24**, 95–112.

Hafner, K.B., Koch, G.G. and Canada, A.T. (1988). Some analysis strategies for three-period changeover designs with two treatments. *Statistics in Medicine*, **7**, 471–82.

Hand, D.J. (1981). *Discrimination and Classification*, Wiley, London.

Hand, D.J. (1985). *Artificial Intelligence and Psychiatry*, Cambridge University Press, Cambridge.

Hand, D.J. (1986). Recent advances in error rate estimation. *Pattern Recognition Letters*, **4**, 335–46.

Hand, D.J. (1992). Statistical methods in diagnosis, *Statistical Methods in Medical Research*, **1**, 49–67.

Hand, D.J. and Taylor, C.C. (1987). *Multivariate Analysis of Variance and Repeated Measures. A Practical Approach for Behavioural Scientists*. Chapman and Hall, London.

Hartigan, J.A. (1975). *Clustering Algorithms*, Wiley, New York.

Hays, W.L. (1963). *Statistics*, Holt, Rinehart and Winston, New York.

Helfenstein, U. (1986). Box–Jenkins modelling of some viral infectious diseases. *Statistics in Medicine*, **5**, 37–48.

Helfenstein, U. (1991). The use of transfer function models, intervention analysis and related time series methods in epidemiology. *International Journal of Epidemiology*, **20**, 808–15.

Helfenstein, U., Achermann-Lubrich, U., Braun-Fahrlander, C. and Wanner, H.U. (1991). Air pollution and diseases of respiratory tracts in pre-school children: a transfer function model. *Journal of Environmental Monitor Assessment*, 17.

Heyting, A., Tolboom, J.T.B.M. and Essers J.G.A. (1992). Statistical handling of dropouts in longitudinal clinical trials. *Statistics in Medicine*, **11**, 2043–

62.
Hill, Bradford A. and Doll, R. (1954). The mortality of doctors in relation to their smoking habits. A preliminary report, *British Medical Journal*, **1**, 1451–5.

Hill – see also under Bradford Hill.

Hills, M. and Armitage, P. (1979). The two period crossover clinical trial. *British Journal of Clinical Pharmacology*, **8**, 7–20.

Hole, D.J., Gullis, G.R., Chopra, C. and Hawthorne, V.M. (1989). Passive smoking and cardio-respiratory health in a general population in the west of Scotland, *British Medical Journal*, **299**, 423–7.

Holford, T.R., White, C. and Kelsey, J.T. (1978). Multivariate analysis for matched case-control studies. *American Journal of Epidemiology*, **107**, 245–56.

Holmquist, N.D., McMahon, C.A. and Williams, O.D. (1967). Variability in classification of carcinoma in situ of the uterine cervix. *Archives of Pathology*, **84**, 334–45.

Huba, G.J., Wingard, J.A. and Bentler, P.M. (1981). A comparison of two latent variable causal models for adolescent drug use. *Journal of Personality and Social Psychology*, **40**, 180–93.

Hunter, K.R., Stern, G.M., Laurence, D.R. and Armitage, D. (1970). Armantradine in Parkinsonism. *Lancet,* **1**, 1127–9.

Huynh, H. and Feldt, L.S. (1976). Estimation of the Box correction for degrees of freedom from sample data in randomized block and split-plot designs. *Journal of Educational Statistics*, **1**, 69–82.

Iles, T.C. (1993) Multiple regression. In *Biological Data Analysis: A Practical Approach*, J.C. Fry (Ed.), Oxford University Press, Oxford.

Iversen, L., Sabroe, S. and Damsgaard, M.T. (1989). Hospital admissions before and after shipyard closure. *British Medical Journal*, **299**, 1073–6.

Jenkins, C.M. and Watts, D.G. (1968). *Spectral Analysis and its Application*, Holden Day, London.

Johnstone, E.C., Lawler, P. and Stevens, M. (1980). The Northwick Park electroconvulsive therapy trial. *Lancet*, **ii**, 1317–20.

Jolliffe, I.T. (1972). Discording variables in a principal component analysis 1: Artificial Data. *Applied Statistics*, **21**, 160–73.

Jolliffe, I.T. (1986). *Principal Component Analysis*, Springer-Verlag, New York.

Jolliffe, I.T. and Morgan, B.J.T. (1992). Principal component analysis and exploratory factor analysis. *Statistical Methods in Medical Research*, **1**, 69–95.

Jones, B. and Kenward, M.G. (1989). *Designs and Analysis of Crossover Trials*, Chapman and Hall, London.

Kalbfleisch, J.D. and Prentice, R.L. (1980). *The Statistical Analysis of Failure Time Data*, Wiley, New York.

Kaplan, E.L. and Meier, P. (1958). Nonparametric estimation from incomplete observations. *Journal of the American Statistical Association*, **53**, 457–81.

Kaprio, J. and Koskenvuo, M. (1988). A prospective study of psychological and socioeconomic characteristics, health behaviour and morbidity in cigarette smokers prior to quitting compared to persistent smokers and non-smokers. *Journal of Clinical Epidemiology*, **41**, 139–50.

Kasser, I. and Bruce, R.A. (1969). Comparative effects of aging, and coronary heart disease and submaximal exercise, *Circulation*, **39**, 759–74.

Kay, R. (1984). Goodness of fit methods for the proportional hazards regression model: a review. *Rev. Epidem. et Santé Publ.,* **32**, 185–98.

Kendall, M.G. and Ord, J.K. (1990). *Time-Series*, 3rd edn, Edward Arnold, London.

Kenward, M. and Jones, B. (1987). The analysis of data from 2 × 2 crossover trials with baseline measurements. *Statistics in Medicine,* **6**, 911–26.

Kershner, R.P. and Federer, W.T. (1981). Two treatment crossover designs for estimating a variety of effects. *Journal of the American Statistical Association*, **76**, 612–19.

Koch, G. and Edwards, S. (1988). Clinical efficacy trials with categorical data. in *Biopharmaceutical Statistics for Drug Development,* C.E. Peace (ed). Marcel Dekker Press, New York.

Kraemer, H.C. and Thiemann, S. (1987). *How many subjects? Statistical Power Analysis in Research*, Sage Publications, Beverly Hills.

Krall, J.M., Uthoff, V.A. and Harley, J.B. (1975). A step-up procedure for selecting variables associated with survival. *Biometrics,* **31**, 49–57.

Kronmall, R.A. and Tarter, M. (1974). The use of density estimates based on orthogonal expansions. In *Exploring Data Analysis — The Computer Revolution in Statistics*. W.J. Dixon and W.L. Nicholson (eds), University of California Press, Berkeley.

Krzanowski, W.J. (1977). The performance of Fisher's linear discriminant function under non-optimal conditions. *Technometrics,* **19**, 191–200.

Landis, J.R. and Koch, G.C. (1977). The measurement of observer agreement for categorical data. *Biometrics,* **33**, 159–74.

Laska, E.M., Meisner, M. and Kulsner, H.B. (1983). Optimal crossover designs in the presence of carryover effects. *Biometrics,* **39**, 1089–91.

Lavori, P. (1990). ANOVA, MANOVA, my black hen, comments on repeated measures, *Archives of General Psychiatry,* **47**, 755–78.

Lazarsfeld, P.L. and Henry, N.W. (1968). *Latent Structure Analysis*, McGraw-Hill, Boston.

Leclerc, A., Lucd, D., Lert, F., Chastang, J.F. and Logeay, P. (1988). Correspondence analysis and logistic modelling: complimentary use in the analysis of a health survey among nurses. *Statistics in Medicine,* **7**, 983–95.

Lee, E.T. (1991). *Statistical Methods for Survival Data Analysis*, 2nd Edn, John Wiley, New York.

Lee, Y.J., Ellenberg, J.H., Hirtz, D.G. and Nelson, K.B. (1991). Analysis of clinical trials by treatment actually received: is it really an option? *Statistics in Medicine,* **10**, 1595–605.

Lellouch, J. and Schwartz, D. (1971). L'essai thérapeutique: éthique individuelle ou éthique collective? *Rev. Inst. Int. Statist.,* **39**, 127–36.

Lind, J. (1753). *A Treatise of the Scurvey.* Reprinted 1953. Edinburgh University Press, Edinburgh.

Link, C.L. (1984). Confidence intervals for the survival function using Cox's proportional-hazard model with covariates. *Biometrics,* **40**, 601–10.

Little, R.J.A. and Rubin, D.B. (1987). *Statistical Analysis of Data with Missing Values*. John Wiley, New York.

Litvak, P., Graziano, J.H., Klue, J.K., Popovic, D., Mehmeti, A., Ahmed, G., Shrout, P., Murphy, J., Gashi, E., Haxhiu, R., Rajovic, L., Nenezic, D. and

Stein, Z. (1991). A prospective study of birthweight and length of gestation in a population surrounding a lead smelter in Kosovo, Yugoslavia. *International Journal of Epidemiology*, **20**, 722–28.

Lock, S. (1982). Preface. *In Statistics in Practice*, S.M. Gore and D.G. Altman (eds) British Medical Association, London.

Lovie, P. (1988). BMDPC and SPCC/PC+, *British Journal of Mathematical and Statistical Psychology*, **41**, 151–54.

Lovie, S. (1989). SAS, *British Journal of Mathematical and Statistical Psychology*, **42**, 133–8.

Lovie, P. (1991a). SYSTAT, *British Journal of Mathematical and Statistical Psychology*, **44**, 240–43.

Lovie, P. (1991b). S-PLUS, *British Journal of Mathematical and Statistical Psychology*, **44**, 237–40.

Lovie, P. (1992). MINITAB Release 8 for DOS, *British Journal of Mathematical and Statistical Psychology*, **45**, 337–38.

McCullagh, P. (1980). Regression models for ordinal data. *Journal of the Royal Statistical Society, Series B*, **42**, 109–42.

McKay, R.J. and Campbell, N.A. (1982a). Variable selection techniques in discriminant analysis. I Description. *British Journal of Mathematical and Statistical Psychology*, **35**, 1–29.

McKay, R.J., and Campbell, N.A. (1982b). Variable selection techniques in discriminant analysis. II Allocation. *British Journal of Mathematical and Statistical Psychology*, **35**, 30–41.

McKnight, B. and van den Eeden, S.K. (1993). A conditional analysis for two-treatment multiple period crossover designs with binomial or Poisson outcomes and subjects who drop out. *Statistics in Medicine*, **12**, 825–34.

McLachlan, G.J. and Basford, K.E. (1988). *Mixture Models: Inference and Applications to Clustering*. Marcel Dekker, New York.

McNemar, Q. (1962). *Psychological Statistics* (3rd edn). Wiley, New York.

McPherson, K. (1974). Statistics: the problem of examining accumulating data more than once. *New England Journal of Medicine*, **290**, 501–2.

McPherson, K. (1982). On choosing the number of interim analyses in clinical trials. *Statistics in Medicine*, **1**, 25–36.

Makuch, R.W., Rosenberg, P.S. and Mulshine, J. (1988). Identifying prognostic factors in binary outcome data: an application using liver function tests and age to predict liver metastases. *Statistics in Medicine*, **7**, 843–56.

Mallows, C.L. (1973). Some comments on C_p. *Technometrics*, **15**, 661–75.

Mantel, N. (1966). Evaluation of survival data and two new rank order statistics arising in its consideration. *Cancer Chemotherapy Reports*, **50**, 163–70.

Mantel, N. (1967). Ranking procedures for arbitrarily restricted observations. *Biometrics*, **23**, 65–78.

Mantel, N. and Haenszel, W. (1959). Statistical aspects of the analysis of data from retrospective studies of disease. *Journal of the National Cancer Institute*, **22**, 719–48.

Mardia, K.V., Kent, J.T. and Bibby, J.M. (1979). *Mutivariate Analysis*, Academic Press, London.

Marsh, N. (1991). STATXACT version 1, *British Journal of Mathematical and Statistical Psychology*, **44**, 419–22.

Matthews, J.N.S., Altman, D.G., Campbell, M.J. and Royston, P. (1989). Analysis of serial measurements in medical research, *British Medical Journal*, **300**, 230–35.

Mehta, C.R., Patel, N.R. and Gray, R. (1985). Computing an exact confidence interval for the common odds ratio in several 2×2 contingency tables. *Journal of the American Statistical Association*, **80**, 969–73.

Micciolo, R., Vantini, I., Cavallini, G., Rubello, W., Talamini, G., Benini, L. and Scuro, L.A. (1985). Correspondence analysis in a study of the clinical evolution of uncomplicated chronic relapsing alcoholic pancreatitis. *Statistics in Medicine*, **5**, 303–10.

Miettinen O.S. (1970). Individual matching with multiple controls in the case of all-or-none responses. *Biometrics*, **26**, 339–55.

Milligan, G.W. (1980). An examination of the effect of six types of error perturbation on fifteen clustering algorithms. *Psychometrika*, **45**, 325–42.

Milligan, G.W. and Cooper, M.C. (1985). An examination of procedures for determining the number of clusters in a data set. *Psychometrika*, **50**, 159–79.

Moolgavkar, S.H., Lustbader, E.D. and Venzan, D.J. (1985). Assessing the adequacy of the logistic regression model for matched case-control studies. *Statistics in Medicine*, **4**, 425–35.

Moore, D.H. (1973). Evaluation of five discrimination procedures for binary variables. *Journal of the American Statistical Association*, **68**, 399–404.

Mumford, E., Schlesinger, H.J., Glass, G.V., Patrick, C. and Cuerdon, T. (1984). A new look of evidence about reduced cost of medical utilization following mental health treatment. *American Journal of Psychiatry*, **41**, 1145–58.

Murray, J., Dunn, G., Williams, P. and Tarnopolsky, A. (1981). Factors affecting the consumption of psychotropic drugs. *Psychological Medicine*, **11**, 551–60.

Nelder, J.A. and Wedderburn, R.W.M. (1972). Generalized linear models. *Journal of the Royal Statistical Society, Series A*, **135**, 370–84.

Neter, J.W., Wasserman, W. and Kutner, M.H. (1985). *Applied Linear Statistical Models. Regression, Analysis of Variance and Experimental Designs*, 2nd Edition, Richard Irwin, Inc., Homewood, Illinois.

Neugut, A.I., Fink, D.J. and Radin, D. (1989). Serum cholesterol and primary brain tumours: a case-control study. *International Journal of Epidemiology*, **18**, 798–801.

Newell, D.J. (1992). Intention-to-treat analysis: implications for quantitative and qualitative research. *International Journal of Epidemiology*, **21**, 837–41.

Oakes, M. (1986). *Statistical Inference: a commentary for the social and behavioural sciences*, Wiley, Chichester.

Oakes, M. (1993). The logic and role of meta-analysis in clinical research. *Statistical Methods in Medical Research*, **2**, 147–60.

Patel, H.I. (1983). Use of baseline measurements in the two period crossover designs. *Communications in Statistics — Theory and Methodology*, **12**, 2693–712.

Patel, M., Gutzwiller, F., Paccaud, F. and Marazzi, A. (1989). A meta-analysis of acupuncture for chronic pain. *International Journal of Epidemiology*, **18**, 900–06.

Paykel, E.S. (1971). Classification of depressed patients: a cluster analysis derived grouping. *British Journal of Psychiatry*, **118**, 275–88.

Paykel, E.S. (1972). Depressive typologies and response to amitryptiline. *British Journal of Psychiatry*, **120**, 147–56.

Paykel, E.S. and Rassaby, E. (1978). Classification of suicide attempters by cluster analysis. *British Journal of Psychiatry*, **133**, 45–52.

Peduzzi, P., Detre, K., Wittes, J. and Holford, T. (1991). Intent-to-treat analysis and the problems of crossovers. An example from the Veterans Administration coronary bypass surgery study. *Journal of Thoracic and Cardiovascular Surgery*, **101**, 481–7.

Peto, R. (1987). Discussion contribution to Light, R.J. *Statistics in Medicine*, **6**, 221–8.

Peto, R. and Peto, J. (1972). Asymptomatically efficient rank invariant procedures *Journal of the Royal Statistical Association, Series A*, **135**, 185–207.

Pickering, G.W. (1949). The place of the experimental method in medicine. *Proceedings of the Royal Society of Medicine*, **42**, 229–34.

Pickering, R.M. and Forbes, J.F. (1984). A classification of Scottish infants using latent class analysis. *Statistics in Medicine*, **3**, 249–51.

Pocock, S.J. (1976). The combination of randomized and historical controls in clinical trials. *Journal of Chronic Disorders*, **29**, 175–88.

Pocock, S.J. (1978). The size of cancer clinical trials and stopping rules. *British Journal of Cancer*, **38**, 757–66.

Pocock, S.J. (1983). *Clinical Trials: A Practical Approach*, Wiley, New York.

Pregibon, D. (1981). Logistic regression diagnostics. *Annals of Statistics*, **9**, 705–24.

Rasmussen, B.K. and Olesen, J. (1992). Symptomatic and nonsymptomatic headaches in a general population. *Neurology*, **42**, 1225–31.

Redmond, A. (1977). *EEG Information, a Didactic Review and Applications*, North Holland, Amsterdam.

Robins, J., Breslow, N. and Greenland, S. (1986). Estimates of the Mantel–Haenszel variance consistent in both sparse data and large-strata limiting model. *Biometrics*, **42**, 311–24.

Römelsjö, A. (1989). The relationship between alcohol consumption and social statistics in Stockholm. Has the social pattern of alcohol consumption changed? *International Journal of Epidemiology*, **18**, 842–51.

Rosenthal, R. (1979). The 'file drawer' and tolerance for null results. *Psychological Bulletin*, **86**, 638–41.

Rozenboom, W.W. (1960). The fallacy of the null hypothesis significance test. *Psychological Bulletin*, **57**, 416–28.

Sacks, H.S., Chalmers, T.C. and Smith, H. (1983). Sensitivity and specificity of clinical trials: randomized vs historical controls. *Archives of Internal Medicine*, **143**, 753–75.

Sartwell, P.E., Masi, A.T., Arthes, F.G., Greene, G.R. and Smith, M.E. (1969). Thromboembolism and oral contraceptives: an epidemiologic case control study. *American Journal of Epidemiology*, **90**, 365–75.

Schouten, H.J.A. (1985). *Statistical Measurement of Interobserver Agreement*. Unpublished doctoral dissertation. Erasmus University, Rotterdam.

Schuster, A. (1898). On the investigation of hidden periodicities. *Terr. Mag.*, **3**, 13.

Senie, R.T., Rosen, P.P., Lesser, M.L. and Kinne, D.W. (1981). Breast self-examination and medical examination related to breast cancer stage,

American Journal of Public Health, 583–90.
Shaw, L.W. and Chalmers, T.C. (1970). Ethics in co-operative clinical trials. *Annals of New York Academy of Science*, **169**, 487–95.
Shortliffe, E.H. (1976). *Computer Based Medical Consultations: MYCIN*, Elsevier, New York.
Simes, R.J. (1987). Confronting publication bias: a cohort design for meta-analysis. *Statistics in Medicine*, **6**, 11–30.
Sinclair, H.M. (1951). Nutritional surveys of population groups. *New England Journal of Medicine*, **245**, 39–47.
Skipper, J.K., Guenther, A.L. and Nass, G. (1967). The sacredness of 0.05: a note concerning the use of statistical levels of significance in social science. *The American Sociologist*, **1**, 16–18.
Sneath, P.H.A. and Sokal, R.R. (1973). *Numerical Taxonomy*, Freeman, San Francisco.
Somes, G.W. and O'Brian, K.F. (1985). Mantel–Haenszel Statistic. In S. Kotz, N.L. Johnson and C.B. Read (eds), *Encyclopedia of Statistical Sciences*, Vol. 5, Wiley, New York.
Sörborm, D. (1978). An alternative to the methodology for analysis of covariance. *Psychometrika*, **43**, 381–96.
Spicer, C.C., Lawrence, C.J. and Southall, D.P. (1987). Statistical analysis of heart rates in subsequent victims of sudden infant death syndrome. *Statistics in Medicine*, **6**, 159–66.
Spiegelhalter, D.J. and Knill-Jones, R.P. (1984). Statistical and knowledge-based approaches to clinical decision-support systems with an application to gastroenterology. *Journal of the Royal Statistical Society, Series A*, **147**, 35–77.
Sprent, P. (1970). Some problems of statistical consultancy. *Journal of the Royal Statistical Society, Series A*, **133**, 139–65.
Sturt, E. (1981). Computerised construction in Fortran of a discriminant function for categorical data. *Applied Statistics*, **30**, 313–25.
Therneau, T.M. (1991). S-PLUS, *American Statistician*, **44**, 239–41.
Therneau, T.M., Grambsch, P.M. and Fleming, T.R. (1990). Martingale based residuals for survival models. *Biometrika*, **77**, 147–60.
Thomas, D.C. (1981). General relative-risk models for survival time and matched case-control studies. *Biometrics*, **37**, 673–86.
Thompson, S.G. (1993). Controversies in meta-analysis: the case of the trials of serum cholesterol reduction. *Statistical Methods in Medical Research*, **2**, 173–92.
Truett, J., Cornfield, J. and Kanel, W. (1967). A multivariate analysis of the risk of coronary heart disease in Framingham. *Journal of Chronic Diseases*. **20**, 511–24.
Tsouros, A.D. and Young, R.J. (1986). Applications of time series analysis: a case study on the impact of computer tomography, *Statistics in Medicine*, **5**, 593–606.
Turner, S.W., Toone, B.K. and Brett-Jones, J.R. (1986). Computerized tomographic scan changes in early schizophrenia — preliminary findings. *Psychological Medicine*, **16**, 219–25.
Umen, A.S.J. and Le, C.T. (1986). Prognostic factors, models and related statistical problems in the survival of end-stage renal disease patients on

hemodialysis. *Statistics in Medicine*, **5**, 637–52.

Upton, G.J.G. (1978). *The Analysis of Cross-Tabulated Data*, Wiley, New York.

Van der Heijden, P.G.M., de Falguerolles, A. and de Leeuw, J. (1989). A combined approach to contingency table analysis using correspondence analysis and loglinear analysis (with discussion). *Applied Statistics*, **38**, 249–92.

Vessey, M.D. and Doll, R. (1969). Investigation of relations between use of oral contraceptives and thromboembolic disease: a further report. *British Medical Journal*, **2**, 651–7.

Ward, J.H. (1963). Hierarchical grouping to optimize an objective function. *Journal of the American Statistical Association*, **58**, 236–44.

Wastell, D.G. (1985). The question of ERP structure: making out the 'figure in the carpet'. In D. Papakostopoulos, S. Butler and I. Martin (eds). *Clinical and Experimental Neurophysiology*, Croom Helm, London.

Wastell, D.G. and Gray, R. (1987). The numerical approach to classification: a medical application to develop a typology for facial pain. *Statistics in Medicine*, **6**, 137–64.

White, S.J. (1979). Statistical errors in papers in the British Journal of Psychiatry. *British Journal of Psychiatry*, **135**, 336–42.

Whittick, J.E. (1989). Dementia and mental handicap: attitudes, emotional distress and caregiving. *British Journal of Medical Psychology*, **62**, 181–9.

Willan, A. and Pater, J. (1986). Carryover and the two-period crossover clinical trial. *Biometrics*, **42**, 593–9.

Winer, B.J. (1971). *Statistical Principles in Experimental Design*, McGraw-Hill, Tokyo.

Wolfe, J.H. (1970). Pattern clustering by multivariate mixture analysis. *Multivariate Behavioural Research*, **5**, 529–50.

Wong, M.A., Sheldon, S. and Olshen, R. (1983). Statistical analysis of gait patterns of persons with cerebral palsy. *Statistics in Medicine*, **2**, 345–54.

Woolson, R.F. and Lachenbruch, P. (1982). Regression analysis of matched case-control data. *American Journal of Epidemiology*, **115**, 444–52.

Yusuf, S., Peto, R., Lewis, J., Collins, R. and Sleight, P. (1985). Beta blockade during and after myocardial infarction. An overview of randomized trials. *Progress in Cardiovascular Disease*, **27**, 335–71.

Index